MEET YOUR
RUNNING GOALS:
HOW NOT TO HATE THE TREADMILL!

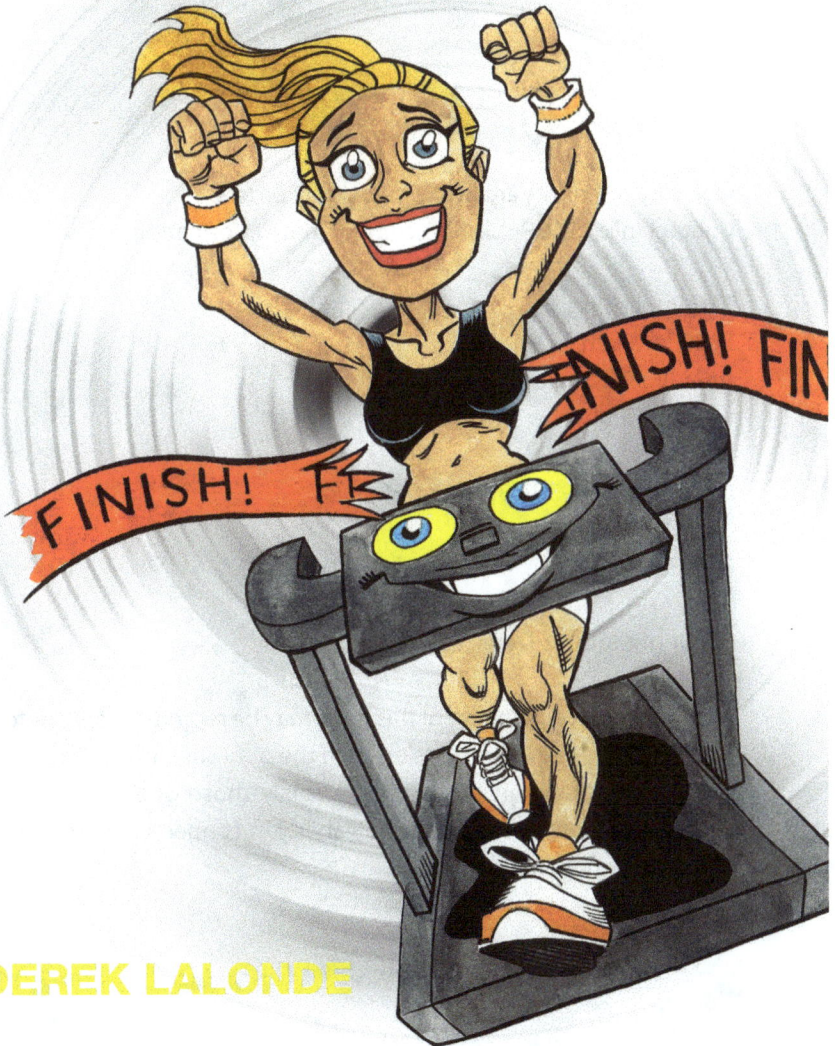

DEREK LALONDE

TAG

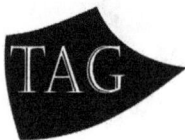

Quantity discounts are available on bulk orders.
Contact info@TAGPublishers.com for more information.

TAG Publishing, LLC
2030 S. Milam
Amarillo, TX 79109
www.TAGPublishers.com

ISBN: 978-1-59930-439-7

First Edition

FOREWORD

I first met Derek in a setting as far as you can get from a basement or health-club treadmill; we were in the Flint Hills of Kansas crewing and pacing his brother to a 100 mile finish.

You might have heard that when it comes to 100 mile races, CREW stands for Cranky Runners, Endless Waiting! So with a lot of time to kill that day, Derek and I talked about various running-related topics. It quickly became clear to me how passionate Derek was about sharing his knowledge with other runners, from novices to the highly competitive. For the last several years, he has educated runners via his website and more recently embarked on a project to help change their attitudes toward treadmills with the development of Treadflix running videos.

Now, Derek has written a book packed with useful information about one of the most misunderstood and under-utilized pieces of exercise equipment, the treadmill. Despite living in the mountains of Colorado with easy access to every kind of terrain imaginable, I myself made treadmill running a key component in my training program, both when training for road races in my twenties, and later as an ultra trail runner. These days, I continue to utilize treadmill training with the runners I coach.The first thing I often hear from runners when talking about treadmills is "I can't run on a treadmill; it is just too boring." And my response is always the same, "that is because you haven't been using it right!" The key to treadmill training is taking advantage of the granular control you have over speed and incline, along with removing the variables of weather, footing, traffic, etc. I purchased my first treadmill when I was working long hours and living at 9000 feet; it was usually dark, icy, or both when I needed to run my workouts.

Over the years, I have found treadmills to be useful in many ways beyond improving fitness. For example, with some minor injuries you can still run or walk uphill on the forgiving surface of your treadmill. It is hard to run uphill only when outside since you need to get back to where you started!

A treadmill is also a great way to work on your running form because you can keep the speed the same while focusing on your stride rate or other components of running form. Filming a runner at different speeds in order to analyze form is much easier on the treadmill than outside.When preparing for his first ultra, a friend of mine even used his treadmill to help determine which was most efficient for him; wearing a camelbak or carrying hand-held water bottles. He did this by running the same pace with each for an hour and comparing his average heart rate. There really is no limit to how you can make use of a treadmill. While you may never come to love running on a treadmill as much as Derek, I can promise you that if you follow his sage advice, you will quickly learn what a powerful tool the treadmill can be in improving as a runner, no matter what type of races you enjoy.

Paul DeWitt
Former Leadville 100 record holder

Running Coach
Palmer Lake, Colorado

www.dewittcoaching.com

DEREK LALONDE

CONTENTS

INTRODUCTION

Waiting. Silent. Still. Eager to hum, spin, grind, flash, run, climb. A partnership bonded by hope, heat, friction, sweat, exhilaration, finish lines. Yearning for contact. Ready to deliver at the touch of a button.

L. Andice

Whether you've already bought a treadmill which is now doubling as a laundry rack, you use a treadmill only reluctantly and every minute feels like as prison sentence, or you are considering the future purchase of a treadmill – this book is for you!

So many people are quick to put down and explain how much they really loathe running on what they commonly refer to as the 'dreadmill'. I get it. I *used* to feel that way.

There really is no point in comparing running on the treadmill to running in nature which offers the possibility of beautiful sights, sounds and smells. Or even make the argument that running on a treadmill could replace experiencing the sense of community, energy and camaraderie that exists while running amongst masses of fellow runners during an organized event.

However, the truth is that in their own category, treadmills are really amazing and effective training tools that can help to change your life and meet your goals. With the offering of un-matched convenience, unbiased work effort, mental training for your mind and body, access to amenities and fuel, the safety of a controlled environment, and many other pluses, it is easy to see that it's worth taking the time to learn how to love the treadmill.

My relationship with the treadmill began 15 years ago when I decided to train for my first marathon. With a gym located close to work, doing a few runs a week on the treadmill became a balance with my outdoor runs. Particularly during the winter months up in Northern Ontario when the temperature with wind chill frequently gets down to minus 30 Celsius. Over the next decade while continuing to set goals and train for runs of various distances, I found myself needing to run more and more but as with most people, my life just seemed to get busier. Purchasing a treadmill for my home then became a great convenience and over a period of 6 years, 85% or more of my weekly training miles were done on the treadmill.

Sometimes this added up to 85 miles a week so I'll be the first to admit that I just had to find a way to **enjoy this time** which had become my reality in chasing my goals as it made no sense to train in ice and snow and be miserable. And then, it finally happened! I actually grew to a point where I looked forward to my treadmill experiences and they became enjoyable.

When I look back to understand how I went from hating to adoring the treadmill, I realized that it wasn't something that happened over night but rather slowly over time. Through the application of many small changes in my environment and awareness of how to leverage the treadmill properly, my paradigm about the treadmill shifted dramatically.

Your ability, or inability, to enjoy training on the treadmill has a heck of a lot to do with your outlook and attitude! Just like any other aspect of your life, if you focus on what you're missing you're going to be cranky. If, however, you can learn how to reverse this attitude you will have completely different treadmill running experiences.

Why should you care about learning to love the treadmill?

Steve Vai, a visionary and brilliant guitarist once said during an interview "Your level of success in the things that you do are a direct reflection of the focus that you have given to those things". Being successful in meeting your goals will require smart and *consistent* training. Learning how to adopt a positive attitude toward the training process **using the treadmill as a tool** will greatly increase your chances of returning for the next workout regardless of the existence of excuses that might otherwise prevent you from doing so.

Over the last 15 years I have gradually learned to love running on the treadmill. And for this, I recognize that I may be a bit out of the norm. While I thoroughly enjoy my time on the treadmill, I never dreamed of writing a book about it. Nor did I think there would be much interest.

That is until about 3 years ago when I noticed a large majority of inquiries on my website (www.meet-your-running-goals.com) started to pour in regarding the struggles many people have with training on treadmills. From these questions and comments coming from runners of ALL levels around the planet, I have come to two conclusions about the large majority of people who do some or much treadmill training.

The first conclusion is actually a misconception, and this is that runners feel treadmill training is less effective at preparing you for your running goals. *I generally get this sense more from beginner runners.*

The second conclusion is that a very large number of runners merely tolerate running on treadmills for the trade-off of conveniences they bring. In fact, I'm pretty sure I've seen every combination of ***negative*** words possible in a sentence used to describe how many people feel about dealing with the boredom of running on treadmills.

It really doesn't have to be this way. In fact, treadmills are awesome and obedient training partners.

Therefore, my goal in writing this book is to show you how, through many small and inexpensive strategies, you can learn to transform your time spent on the treadmill from tolerance to enjoyment.

These findings were also a huge inspiration that led to the creation of **Treadflix.com** which provides runners (including myself) fun, interactive and effective training videos to use on the treadmill. In addition to gaining some value from this book, I am also hopeful that you will explore some of these videos I and my team at **TreadFlix.com** have worked hard to bring to life for your enjoyment and training benefit!

The late Earl Nightingale once said: "***We are at our very best, and we are happiest, when we are fully engaged in work we enjoy on the journey toward the goal we've established for ourselves.***"

I look forward to every single opportunity to run on a treadmill, and I hope this book will help you to enjoy the training journey too!

DEREK LALONDE

TREADMILL BENEFITS – SOME FACTS!

No matter what distance you're training for, there is quite an extensive list of benefits that runners (and walkers) of all levels can take advantage of. Coupled with a handful of simple strategies that I'll reveal to you later in the book, you'll be on your way to leveraging this powerful training tool.

Let's start by increasing your awareness of what treadmills have to offer because they do, in fact, offer countless conveniences and training benefits to runners (and walkers) of all levels. Perhaps there are a good number of benefits listed here that you had not previously considered.

Forgiving Running Surface

Gerry hasn't been running for 7 years since his last corporate 5k. His hectic work travel schedule, busy family life, love for good food and lack of clear running goals have all taken their toll on his body. For over a year now Gerry has been thinking about getting back into running especially as he drives by runners out there pounding the pavement after a long day at work.

Finally, on one bright Saturday morning, the fuel and spark come together to ignite his motivation to get out the door for a run. He quickly gathers what workout clothes he can put together. His running gear happens to include an old pair of trail shoes that he purchased about 7 years back. *Good enough,* he thinks and off he goes out the front door, down the street and down the sidewalk for the 6 mile route he used to run back in the day.

It sure took a while for the heart, lungs and legs to all come together. In fact, the first 15 minutes were incredibly discouraging. However, eventually, that long lost inner running partner returned and by the time he reached the 3 mile turnaround he was feeling fantastic!

One mile later, with 2 miles left to get back home, he was feeling the pain of his weight gain and long lay-off in his knees and lower back. *I can't stop now,* he thought. *Gotta get home!* With dogged determination he ground out the last 2 miles home.

The next day, Gerry's lower back and knees were in such bad shape he had trouble bearing weight on them. Maybe he went too far too soon. Maybe it was the worn out cross trainers or perhaps the unforgiving surface of the sidewalk.

For someone like Gerry who's been on the couch for a while looking to get back into running, treadmills provide an amazing ability to absorb a large amount of ground contact force. While they certainly don't take the place of running with good form, they do help to dissipate this force down through the deck sparing the runner some unnecessary and undue damage to joints, muscles and back. This is an important feature particularly if the body is not accustomed to running after a lay off. Had Gerry opted for a hop on the treadmill to get back into running, he would have had the option to hop off at mile 4 when his body was giving him strong signals that a threshold had been reached and he was doing damage by pushing too hard.

The absorption feature of treadmills not only helps newer runners re-integrate from a long lay-off, but it also helps more advanced runners needing to log some serious high mileage weeks during marathon (or ultra-marathon) training without getting injured.

Accomplished ultra-runner Paul DeWitt (**Dewittcoaching.com**), lives and trains amongst some of the most beautiful and rugged trail systems in the world. To compliment his high mileage training and help stay off the injury list, Paul has always regularly incorporated a good amount of his weekly training on the treadmill. Furthermore, he also prescribes much of the same for many of his clients who train to meet their marathon and longer distance goals.

So the forgiving responsiveness of the running deck is, without a doubt, high on the list of benefits that treadmills provide to the widest range of runners. From runners getting back at it after a long lay-off to advanced distance runners looking to log high mileage weeks and stay off the injury list.

Treadmills also provide the following list of benefits for runners and walkers alike:

- Effective **group runs** for different levels – running with others can be awesome but individuality is accompanied by different fitness levels. Running side by side on treadmills at the gym is a great way to run with a partner while each runner or walker gets the workout that serves them best without compromising the other.

- Good practice for running **cadence** – since treadmills offer consistent speed and digital time readouts, it's easy to perform cadence drills such as 'quick feet' to work on your leg turn over speed.

- **Change your course** and challenge at the touch of a button – treadmills offer all of the dynamics of a training program from a recovery run to hill runs and all the way up to blistering speed sessions all at the touch of a button.

- **Safe environment** – no dangerous traffic, dogs or fear of running in the dark. Terry lives in Kenner, LA. She loves to run and she's training to do her 3rd marathon. She prefers running outside but, unfortunately, her schedule can get pretty hectic and so often the only time she has left to train is after dark. Neither Terry nor her husband are comfortable with her running through the neighborhoods in the dark, so the treadmill has become an invaluable ally in getting ready for her next race.

- Treadmills can offer a very **entertaining and motivating** environment (*see Motivation chapter!*).

- **Easy access to fuel** – anyone who has marathon trained on a point to point course knows the logistics involved with making fuel drop arrangements. Not only does having your fuel next to you save time, it allows you to practice drinking at 'race pace' which will come in handy on the day of your event.

- Easy **access to bathroom** facilities.

- **Great mental training** – for focus and heart rate control – treadmills provide mental training in a wide variety of ways including teaching you how to focus and have patience. Learning how to relax and bring your heart rate down while you're exercising is one of the most powerful skills you can acquire.

- Excellent tool for the safe and gradual **transition to minimalist/barefoot running**.

- Home treadmills provide the opportunity for **visits from the family** – what a great perk to have one of your family members come for a visit while you're working out! I also get frequent visits from my two Vizslas. They are not big fans of my treadmill.

- **Electrolyte management** - as a profuse sweater, I would like to highlight that treadmill running indoors is excellent training for electrolyte loss management. In fact, many runners get all of the factors right when preparing for race day *except* this. This is particularly true for home gyms without central air managing the air temperature in the room of your treadmill.

Once running in the dead of winter when it was -32C outside, I noticed that the air in my basement workout room was a crisp 17C when I started. Forty-five minutes into the run, the air exchanger pipes running through the uncovered ceiling above my treadmill started to drip. The motor of the treadmill created enough heat to raise the temperature of the room by about 5 degrees. It stands to reason that the most direct temperature change will be felt by the runner who is only a few feet from the treadmill motor. Even commercial motors will produce some heat during operation.

Many experienced runners can attest to the value of learning how to stay in control of your fluid and electrolyte levels in order to ensure success during your running events.

On the other end of the spectrum, even if your room is on the warm or cool side, running indoors can often offer a superior training experience compared to running in some of the temperature extremes many runners face in other parts of the world.

In the extreme heat in some places like Texas, you may be forced to drastically slow your pace and maybe even cut your run short to avoid the dangers of depletion and heat stroke. In the extreme cold of Northern Ontario, it can get to a point where you are wearing so many layers you feel like you are running in a scuba suit. Not to mention trying to breathe naturally through an ice crusted face mask.

While braving the elements can be an adventure, and you'll definitely rack up tough guy points, sometimes you've got to be honest with yourself about the real training benefits of what you're doing and look for a better way.

- **Consistent Speed training** - there are several types of workouts where having a consistent belt speed provides a very advantageous training benefit. Out on the track a runner will perform repeats of say 10 x 800 meters. The last few repeats may be a little slower as the runner tires or a bit quicker as the runner digs deep to make the end of the workouts really count. The treadmill, once set at a determined speed, will require the runner to stay focussed in order to keep up with the belt regardless of how the runner 'feels' about the situation. Digging deep is still possible by quickly reaching up and hitting the speed increase arrow but otherwise the goal pace must be maintained.

During some harder lactate training sessions where you are staying at, or around, a specific heart rate for prolonged periods, having the ability to set the treadmill speeds is invaluable. The runner can focus on breathing and good form without having to continually check heart rate. The instant incline option is also a great feature to increase one's heart rate without having to speed up.

Treadmills have the following shortfall:

- **Lack of Specificity** for Road Running – despite the long list of positive features that do exist on treadmills to get you ready for your running event, you are in fact training in a controlled environment. Race day will bring hard ground and can bring some interesting weather.

With this in mind, while the majority of your training runs can be completed on the treadmill, try your best to get some of your runs done outside with similar terrain to your event. Not only will the terrain vary, but your legs and lungs will receive quite a shock when you hit the pavement outside. It is unrealistic to expect your body to do well without that controlled air and belt turning under your feet. Later in the chapter on running form, I go into a little more detail about the differences of running over ground versus on a moving belt.

The bottom line is that while treadmills don't **completely** replace running outdoors they are phenomenal training tools to help you reach your goals. So any runner would be amiss if they thought otherwise

DEREK LALONDE

IS TREADMILL RUNNING HARDER OR EASIER THAN RUNNING OUTSIDE?

One would think the answer to this question was a simple **yes or no**; however the truth can be as subjective as a person's taste in music! It all depends on how a person defines easy or hard. Physiologically, it's possible to prove that running 7 miles/hour on the treadmill is easier or harder than a given similar outside route by co-relating heart rates; however, there are many factors that play into the equation.

For example, while the treadmill may be in a controlled environment, an unconditioned room that averages 70 degrees Fahrenheit will actually increase in temperature as the treadmill runs causing the runner to perspire which will have a direct impact on the runner's heart-rate. Inversely, an outdoor run in cooler temperatures on a flat course such as a track may actually produce a lower heart rate and therefore be considered 'easier' than the treadmill at an equivalent pace.

Some runners find the treadmill much more **mentally** challenging than running outside due to the lack of stimulation – as in smells, sights and sounds. While it's easy to chalk this up as a downside, training in these types of monotonous conditions can actually help a great deal to build mental toughness for a runner. Particularly for longer events like marathons and beyond where there will inevitably be prolonged moments of discomfort and possibly loneliness. If you're used to finding ways to occupy your mind during these miles you'll obviously fare much better than those who are not.

However, it's the monotony of running on a treadmill that also helps build mental toughness for those longer events.

Physically, there is good argument both for and against the treadmill with its lack of variation in terrain. Some runners would find the surface easier to handle due to the slight absorption of the deck where others would argue that a lack of terrain dynamics causes specific muscle fatigue due to the repetitive and consistent nature.

Inclines can be simulated as with running outside on a hilly course however most treadmills don't typically come with a decline feature. As you'll see later in the book however, this is an obstacle that is quite easily and inexpensively overcome!

As mentioned above, another very powerful argument for treadmills is they can often provide a much better specific training workout when the weather is inclement. Especially if braving the elements means running in biting winds, snow and perhaps less than desirable footing. Between layering and less than adequate footing, you may be left with logging some junk miles at best when compared to being able to keep a quicker steady pace in a controlled setting.

You no doubt will build memories, gain bragging rights and even score some macho points with fellow runners if you choose to run in the ice and snow, but you're not necessarily preparing yourself better for your upcoming run.

At the end of the debate, by far the most important thing to determine is whether or not the treadmill is going to properly **prepare you for the demands of the running event you are training for**!

As far as research with empirical data analyzing this question, there are several studies including one particularly interesting one performed by Jack Daniels (the physiologist, not the whiskey maker). Dr. Daniels looked to provide objective scientific proof to support or negate the claim that treadmill running was easier than running outside. Furthermore, this data was useful to runners all over the world who are interested to know if they are properly preparing for an event by doing their runs on a treadmill. The main variable between the two environments, for the purpose of the study, was the possible factor of wind resistance a runner may encounter while running outside on a flat surface versus the lack of wind resistance on a treadmill.

Using this difference in wind resistance on a runner outdoors versus indoors, he was able to determine which grade on the treadmill would create an equivalent effort. The study finds that the faster one runs, the greater a factor that wind resistance becomes… but only to a point. Below a pace of 8 miles per hour on the treadmill, the lack of wind resistance is barely measureable and therefore negligible as far as registering an impact on the energy/effort demands of the runner.

In summary, if you're running 8 mph or more, increase the treadmill to 1% grade to get the equivalent training as an outdoor flat course and to aid with a slight body lean for good running form; otherwise you can leave it at 0%.

MOTIVATION

While the focus of this book is most certainly about the many ways there are to increase your enjoyment of working out on the treadmill, at the core is something that is absolutely fundamental to trigger human action of any kind. It is the single driver and spark responsible for the tackling of any endeavour that you may embark on in your life: Motivation!

Getting your butt on the treadmill day after day to succeed at meeting your running goals requires a combination of the following elements:

4 Pillars of Motivation

- *Great Goals*
- *Positive Environment*
- *Stimulating Activities*
- *Positive Results*

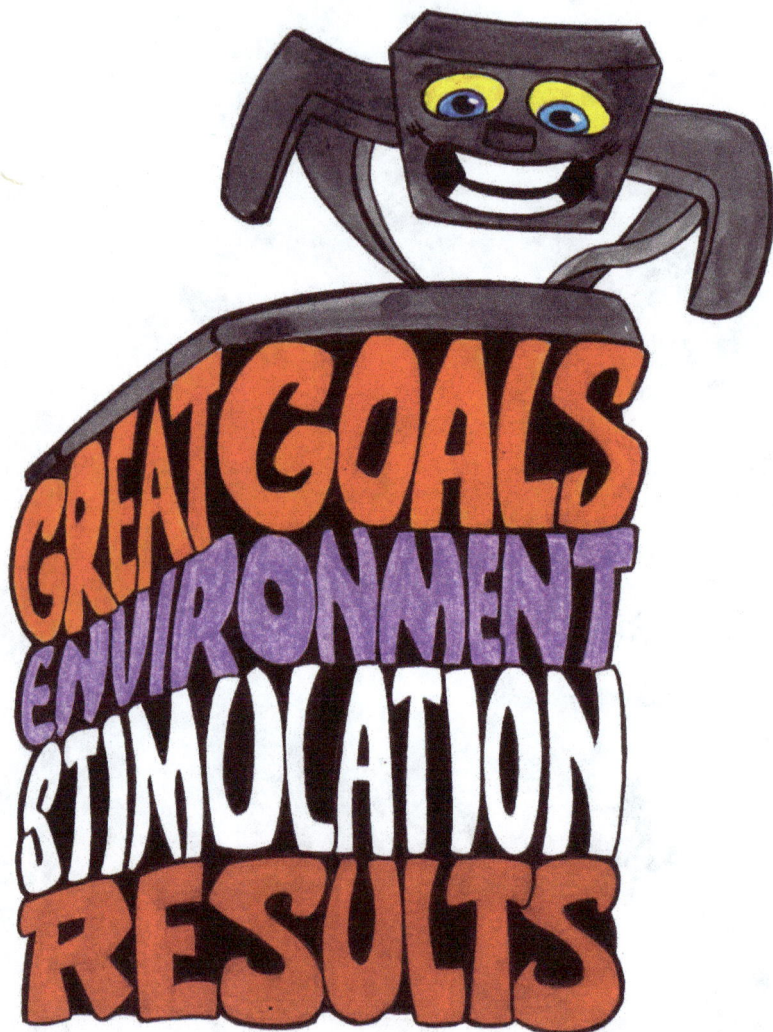

GREAT GOALS
ENVIRONMENT
STIMULATION
RESULTS

·A·

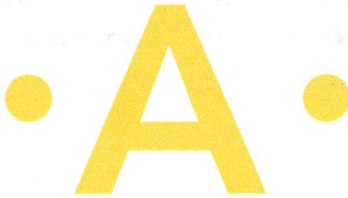

SET GREAT GOALS

Why are goals so important for motivation? While motivation is the spark, your clearly defined goals are the fuel that stokes the fire of action!

Setting and achieving the right short-term goals gives you a clear destination. They are encouraging, motivating and positive signs of forward progress toward your longer term goals.

Setting the right goals is the foundation for your motivation to exercise on a consistent basis whether it's on the treadmill or not!

It's really worth taking the time to properly learn how to set goals that are right for you and that you have a good shot at meeting if you apply yourself.

One of the best goal setting strategies that anyone can use to consistently make effective goals involves applying the **SMART** principles to individually tailored goals. The reason for this is goals written in this fashion provide you with a *crystal clear* vision of what it is you want, how you're going to get it and even *when* you're going to get it!

SMART goals are:

1. **S**pecific – "I will run a marathon…" (26.2 miles)
2. **M**easurable – "…within a time of 4 hours, 15 minutes, 30 seconds…"
3. **A**ction oriented – run
4. **R**ealistic yet challenging – last marathon was 4:30:00 (shaving off 14 min./30 seconds)
5. **T**ime or deadline oriented– "…on May 24, 2016".

SMART GOALS FOR RUNNERS

To ensure that you stay motivated throughout your training program and to optimize your chances for success, I recommend that you carve out at least **3** types of goals for yourself including:

1. **Step goals**
2. **Program goals**
3. **Career(Ultimate)goals**

Step Goals

These are the short-term stepping stones that keep you motivated and on the right path toward your longer term goals. For example, throughout your program you should have at least a few races planned that you may have specific time goals for. In addition to providing an immediate objective to focus on, short term goals can be very helpful indicators as to your current fitness and hence training program effectiveness. By using a tool such as a pace calculator and race prediction chart, you can plug in some of your race times and obtain some pretty accurate estimates for your bigger goals!

Program Goals

These are the goals that you intend to achieve at the end of any given training program. For example, an average half or full marathon training program may be 18 weeks long which includes a 2 or 3 week taper leading up to a goal race on the final day.

Running Career Goals

Of course, most of us can't make a living from the potential spoils of running races. We do however have long-term running aspirations that we would like to eventually achieve in our running journey! While you may be weeks, months or even years away from your running career goal, it should be a grandiose one. Your career goal can be a specific race time, such as run a half marathon in a time of 1 hour 25 minutes, a sub 3 hour marathon or even a total number of miles that you wish to log in your lifetime such as 40,000 miles. Why not have a few?

Use a tool such as the goal setting worksheet (a downloadable and printable version can be found at **www.meet-your-running-goals/goal-setting-worksheet.html)** and take the time to set your step goals in addition to your program goals so that you have short-term milestones to focus on. It's important that you write out your goals on the goal setting worksheet, and post them in an **obvious** place that you will see, or at least refer to, every day. This is one of the most powerful goal setting strategies you can employ since goals are not much good if they are out of sight and out of mind.

Your goals should be challenging, something you have not achieved already, but also realistic. A goal setting guru by the name of Raymond Aaron wrote in his book, *Double Your Income Doing What you Love*, points out that there is a negative psychological impact when you win by losing.

So, if you purposely set your goals way too high expecting that you'll at least achieve something close to it and expect that you'll be satisfied you'll often find that you're disappointed. He uses the example of 4 teams in the final playoffs playing for medals. There are at last two teams who play for the honour of Bronze and only one of them will win and receive the Bronze medal. The other two teams are playing for Gold and while one team will receive the Silver medal, a higher honour than Bronze, they will only receive the Silver *by losing* while going for Gold!

On the other hand, your big goals should be something that your combined genetics, long term accumulated fitness, focus and hard work will allow you to achieve.

DEREK LALONDE

GOAL SETTING MISTAKES

Along the same vein as setting goals that are completely unrealistic for you, I've often seen runners make the mistake of **being too lackadaisical about what they really want**.

After finishing a local 5k run, Troy stood by watched the half marathon finishers cross the line and got bit by the running bug. He decided he wanted to experience what he saw and started running and training for his first half marathon. He struggled with a bit of extra weight and some ITB issues so he asked me for a bit of help putting together a program to add some structure to his training. When I asked him what his goal for the half marathon was, he looked at me strangely and said "What do you mean? I just want to finish in one piece of course!" Fair enough!

Race day came and Troy's months of training really came together. He ran a smart, patient run and finished strong out on the 'rolling scenic' course. I congratulated him at the finish line and the very first thing that came out of his mouth was "Thanks but I was really hoping to break 2 hours."

While Troy stated he had no specific goal for the half, he did possess a secret goal which robbed him of taking even a brief amount of time to enjoy his accomplishment. The idea of Troy finishing in a time that was just 2 minutes shy of what he really wanted was heartbreaking to him.

Troy's reaction of not being satisfied was not the

problem. There is absolutely nothing wrong with yearning for more and in fact, not being satisfied with your own performance is critical for athletes to accomplish more and push their boundaries.

However, had Troy communicated his secret goal of breaking 2 hours, we could have taken some time to work out a reasonable race plan for the day which would have given him some structure, focus and a greater chance of reaching his goal. It could have been as simple as walking 10 less seconds at each aid station. Even if he had followed a plan and not reached his goal, he could rest easier that he took more than a shot in the dark approach at making it happen.

The good news is Troy's performance provided him a great benchmark for setting his next half marathon goal.

So, if you have a secret goal which is something you really want, at least acknowledge it to yourself, write it down and **develop a pacing plan** accordingly to help yourself succeed on race day.

One other goal setting mistake I've seen quite a few (beginner) runners make is to set **goals that involve placing in the race** based on elements such as overall place, age, gender, etc.

The runs I'm most proud of are those where I know I left nothing in training or on the course that day. Even if I didn't meet my goal that day, if I think I did everything in my power to make it happen then I'm proud of my performance.

I won a half marathon a few years ago which was an incredibly exhilarating and fun experience! I was really proud of myself that day. Not because I was first, but because instead of hanging out and drinking beer by the pool, I chose to show up and then run my ass off to the best of my ability.

I came in first because none of the other faster runners (and there are many) bothered to show up that night. It also happened to be a rather low key run that was unusual in that it started at 7 in the evening on a Saturday! It did get me thinking that I should start looking for the world's most remote and uninteresting runs in the hopes that no other runners would show up and I could claim first again!

You have **NO** control over anything that is outside of your best effort and therefore statements such as "I want to place first in my age group" should not be a part of your goal.

So, while there is always a place for your huge goals, make them your career goals and set your immediate and program goals to carve a path of success that will lead you there, one step at a time.

> **A clearly defined purpose and goal is crucial to remind yourself everyday exactly why you need to get your butt on the treadmill instead of play another round of 'Candy Crush'.**

GOAL SETTING WORKSHEET:

Step\Immediate Goals – *On March 5th I will run the 5k in a time of 21:00*
1
2
3

Current Program Goals – *On August 8th, 2012 I will run the full marathon in a time of 3:15:00*
1
2
3

Career Goals – *I will run the full marathon in under 3 hours. On my 56th birthday, I will have completed 56 half marathons.*
1
2
3

Signature: _____

Current Date: _____

Here's a summary of the top goal setting strategies:

1. **Write your goals down!**

2. **Make sure your goals are smart (the next chapter is about *realistic* goals).**

3. **Create short-term and long-term goals.**

4. **Get emotionally involved with your goals.**

5. **Post your goals in an obvious place.**

A goal setting strategy that works great for me, and many other runners I know, is to plug your goals into a nice large calendar that you can put in your kitchen or bedroom that is on display for you to see and affirm every day.

Whether you use an app or a hard copy printed calendar to follow your running training program, plug in your step goals by writing the exact date that you plan on executing or achieving them. For example, in January if I have a program goal that I plan to run in May then my training program will peak on that day in May. Between January and May, however, I also need step goals to provide me with short-term motivation and focus throughout the long training period. My 2 steps goals could consist of a 10k run in March, and a half marathon goal in April. I will then find races that roughly coincide to a good fit in my 4 month training program and build them in with specific time goals for each that will compliment my program goal.

In summary, when you read your written goals they should excite and maybe even scare you a little(or a lot!). If they do this, you've done a good job of applying sound goal setting strategies since this means you're pushing yourself to progress beyond what is already common to you. Remember, it's important to read your goals frequently, if possible at least once a day, and get emotionally attached to them.

Envision what it will feel like when you achieve them. As you'll notice later in the book, the creation of the running movies on **Treadflix.com** was inspired by the need to visualize and get as emotionally involved with my upcoming goals as possible. Running occasionally, or frequently, to the **Treadflix** videos should prove to be great goal preparation tools if any of your goals include running a major marathon.

HOW TO SET 'REALISTIC GOALS'

If you haven't already done so, the first thing you want to do, is use a race prediction chart and plug in some recent race times. You will be provided with some reasonable estimates for your immediate and step goals (see description that follows). You can also use the pace calculator tool if you need to work out running paces for different event distances based on your desired finished time. This will give you an idea if your goal pace is challenging yet realistic.

Next, when you are thinking about setting your running goals, it's important to consider and have an awareness of your weaknesses and strengths. As any level runner, we have some things that we are good at and things that we can work on or currently struggle with.

Identify your Strengths and Weaknesses

You can identify some of your strengths and weakness by considering the following:

1. **Past successes**

2. **Past failures**

3. **Input of others (qualified coach, mentor, trusted friend/athlete)**

Honesty

After years of trying to qualify for Boston, I would get close qualifying times but seemed to do a little worse in subsequent attempts. One day after a marathon that yielded me what I thought was a less than spectacular attempt, I sat (probably sulking) waiting for a post run massage. I started up a conversation with a fellow runner next to me with a heavy Polish accent who had just run a great marathon time.

Perhaps it was a combination of language barrier and his personality, but he had a very direct way of communicating. When he asked me how I did I told him about my disappointment with my performance that day. He paused for about 5 seconds, looked over at me and said "Well, you'll never run fast eating at McDonald's all the time". I was stunned! I had known this man for under 1 minute and he had the nerve to tell me I was too fat to do well at marathons!

Well of course, he was absolutely right and eventually his abrupt yet sage advice sunk in and I went to work making some changes to help me meet my goals. Ted and I eventually became good friends over the years and many marathons later, after a particularly good run I got a call from him. With his thick Polish accent he said, "There you go. Now you're running fast". I attribute a big part of the progress I made after that day to him.

While it's absolutely essential to believe in yourself and your abilities, realize that it can be difficult to self-coach. You should try to be open to the input of a trusted coach or fellow athlete that knows you and cares about your success, particularly if you are not experiencing much success. They may not always be right, but give any input some careful consideration before dismissing it. For example, if you always fade or get passed going up hills and you will be racing a hilly course, consider more emphasis on hill training for your next program. If you consistently stay on your goal pace until mile 19 and then badly fade, have a good look at the number and length of long runs that you have been doing to prepare for your run.

Setting SMART goals means your goals should be specific, measurable, action-oriented, realistic and time based. Many of these goal elements are easy enough to figure out, if you can first determine **WHAT** it is that constitutes a 'realistic' goal for you.

Never Run a Race Before?

If you are a brand new runner, and you've never actually run any organized road race, or completed any measured distance before, setting smart goals is pretty straight forward. You should aim to finish with no pre-set time goal. There are a couple of reasons for this. Firstly, simply **doing** something that you've never done before is an accomplishment and you should feel the full joy of that. Second, with no previous benchmarks to compare your fitness to, you may either make your goal too challenging or not challenging enough. In either case, you run the risk of taking away from the gratification that you deserve for finishing!

Have a Recent Race Performance?

If you have completed at least one recent past road race of any distance ranging from 5k to the half marathon, you can use the race prediction chart which follows to properly select your next goal.

I created the chart using Peter Reigel's prediction formula (t2 = t1 * (d2 / d1)^1.06) for estimated finishing times of longer distances based on times of previously completed distances. It's useful if you have a recent race time and are looking to pick a good realistic goal for a **longer** distance.

How to use the Chart

The chart contains finishing times for various race distances. Find your most recent race time for a 5k, 10k or half marathon. To find what time you could reasonably expect to run a **longer** distance, follow the row to the right.

For example, let's say that I want to set a SMART goal for a half marathon in the spring. Three months ago, I ran a 5k in a time of 22:25. So I find the nearest time to 22:53 on the chart, which is **23:00**. To see what I should be able to run based on that performance, I follow that row to the right. In this case, I get a goal time of **1:48:32**. You might consider going a bit bigger and dropping a bit of time as well to make sure your goal is challenging and will require you to push your boundaries! You will at least be in the ball park.

Keep in mind that while this forecasted time is a reasonable expectation based on a recent previous performance, it is *assuming the proper training has been completed*. For example, because a 16 year old high school student can run a 17 minute 5k, it does not mean that she can necessarily run a 2:50:00 marathon if she has not done the required endurance based training to allow her to tap into her speed for a prolonged distance. In fact, racing the marathon at a 2:50:00 pace without having done long runs would set this runner up for a very hard and painful lesson not soon forgotten!

Please recognize that this is a prediction formula, based on physiological factors and studies of other runner's equivalent race times - it is not a fortune teller or a guarantee.

Just the same, setting SMART goals by using this chart is a great start to get you on your way to achieving more than you ever thought possible.

RACE PREDICTION CHART

5k Time	10k time	Half Time	Full Time
0:35:00	1:14:12	2:45:10	5:50:09
0:34:30	1:13:08	2:42:48	5:45:09
0:34:00	1:12:04	2:40:27	5:40:09
0:33:30	1:11:01	2:38:05	5:35:09
0:33:00	1:09:57	2:35:43	5:30:08
0:32:30	1:08:54	2:33:22	5:25:08
0:32:00	1:07:50	2:31:00	5:20:08
0:31:30	1:06:46	2:28:39	5:15:08
0:31:00	1:05:43	2:26:17	5:10:08
0:30:30	1:04:39	2:23:55	5:05:08
0:30:00	1:03:36	2:21:34	5:00:08
0:29:30	1:02:32	2:19:12	4:55:08
0:29:00	1:01:28	2:16:51	4:50:07
0:28:30	1:00:25	2:14:29	4:45:07
0:28:00	0:59:21	2:12:08	4:40:07
0:27:30	0:58:18	2:09:46	4:35:07
0:27:00	0:57:14	2:07:24	4:30:07
0:26:30	0:56:10	2:05:03	4:25:07
0:26:00	0:55:07	2:02:41	4:20:07
0:25:30	0:54:03	2:00:20	4:15:06
0:25:00	0:53:00	1:57:58	4:10:06
0:24:30	0:51:56	1:55:37	4:05:06
0:24:00	0:50:52	1:53:15	4:00:06
0:23:30	0:49:49	1:50:53	3:55:06
0:23:00	0:48:45	1:48:32	3:50:06
0:22:30	0:47:42	1:46:10	3:45:06
0:22:00	0:46:38	1:43:49	3:40:05
0:21:30	0:45:34	1:41:27	3:35:05
0:21:00	0:44:31	1:39:06	3:30:05
0:20:30	0:43:27	1:36:44	3:25:05
0:20:00	0:42:24	1:34:22	3:20:05
0:19:30	0:41:20	1:32:01	3:15:05
0:19:00	0:40:16	1:29:39	3:10:05
0:18:30	0:39:13	1:27:18	3:05:05
0:18:00	0:38:09	1:24:56	3:00:04
0:17:30	0:37:06	1:22:35	2:55:04
0:17:00	0:36:02	1:20:13	2:50:04
0:16:30	0:34:58	1:17:51	2:45:04
0:16:00	0:33:55	1:15:30	2:40:04
0:15:30	0:32:51	1:13:08	2:35:04

B

CREATE A POSITIVE ENVIRONMENT

A second really important component to increase your motivation to get on the treadmill (and the heart of this book) is to make sure that you are set up for success. This means take a bit of time to create a workout environment that you will actually *look forward* to spending time in. While these changes certainly do not have to be expensive or time consuming, the results can have a huge impact on your success. It's also definitely the one area that many people fail to take the time to do right and therefore leave little chance of changing their attitude about treadmill running.

So why do so many treadmills become clothes racks in some desolate part of the basement or laundry room?

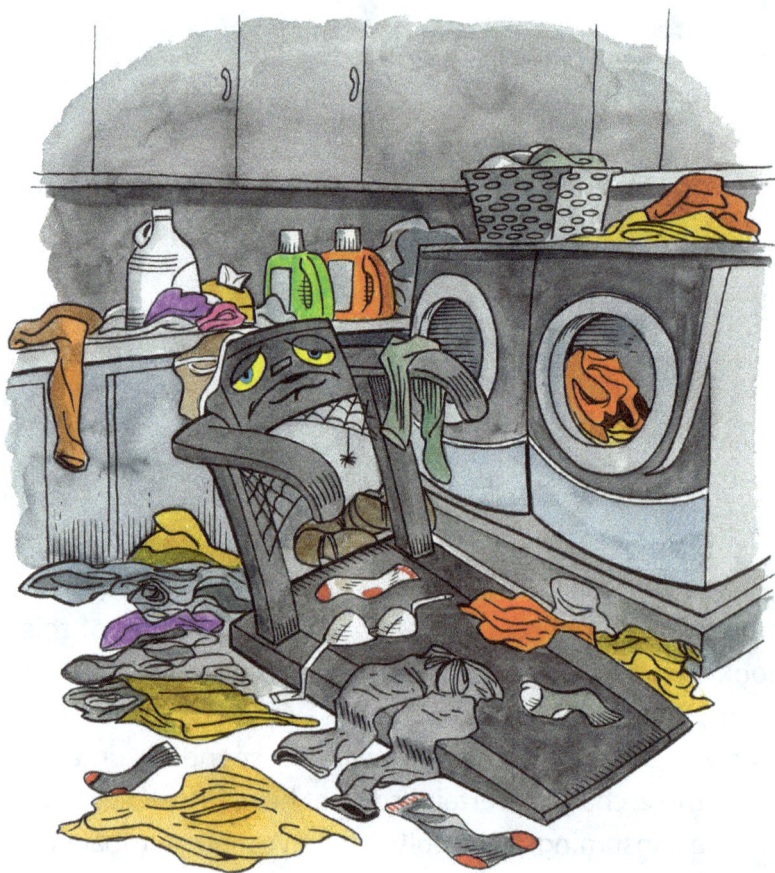

Well, for starters, a cluttered laundry room or dingy unfinished portion of the basement does not usually qualify as a place in your house that you want to spend time in. Unless your goal is to morph into the pink panther, why on earth would you want to stare at this every day for hours on end?

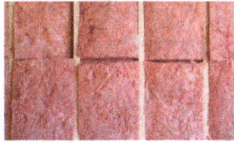

Yet, so many people setup their treadmill in the basement with a similar type of view. Perhaps there's a part of us deep down that knows if it's out of sight, it's out of mind. And boy you would be right! A part of me can't help but wonder if we do this as a subconscious way to create another good excuse to not work out. Nah, that's the **OLD** you!

Motivation starts from the centre of your physical being, your brain. Your motivation to act, or react, in this world toward an end result (goal) is based on your brain's response to the information that surrounds you and that which is taken in by your various **senses** including your sight, smell, hearing, taste and touch.

There's really no argument that running on a treadmill will always be an 'artificial' substitute for running outdoors, which is why it's so important to ensure that your treadmill is situated in an indoor setting that's as positive, enjoyable and stimulating to you as possible. That includes stimulating sights, smells, sounds and feel.

You may have noticed that treadmill advertisements typically show beautiful people, happily running in a well-designed, spacious area complete with vaulted ceilings and gorgeous stone fireplaces. The reason for this is advertisements and commercials are designed to really highlight the 'sizzle' of the product that they are trying to sell, or the dream of what can be if you buy that product. Buy this and you'll look like her and have what she has!

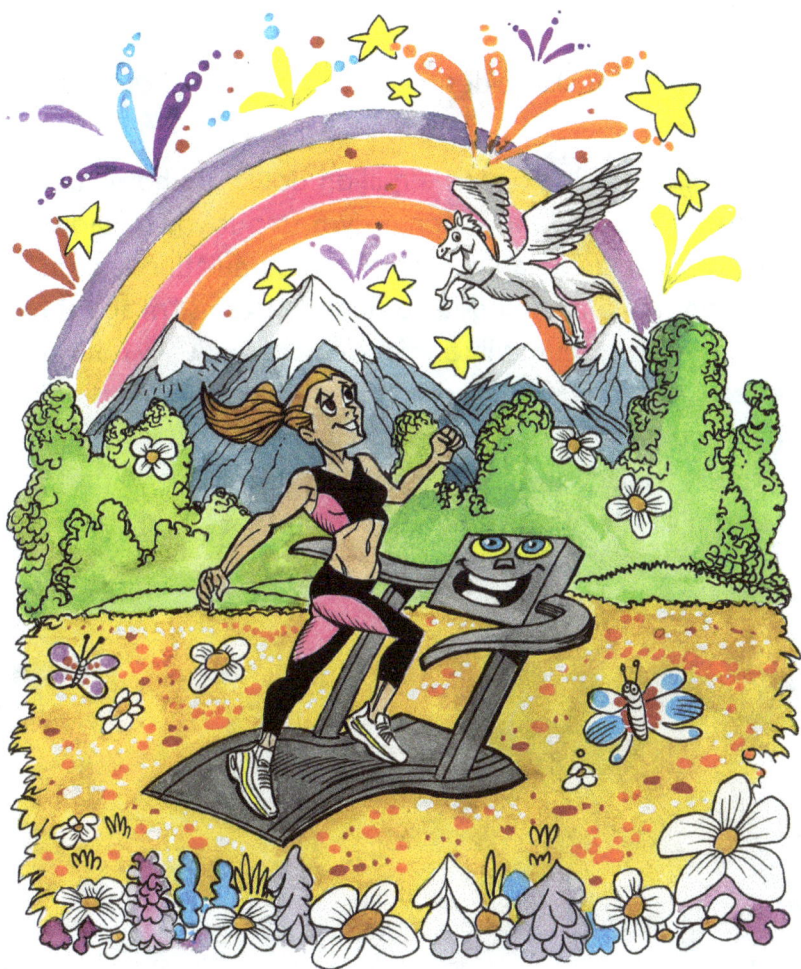

By the same token, big box stores put a lot of thought and energy into the feel of their stores to create an environment that is both inviting and stimulating. Everything from the entrance to the initial feel upon entering the store created by the space and its sights, sounds and smells are designed to motivate visitors to stay and shop.

While you don't need a million dollar log home from Aspen complete with a home gym to put your treadmill in, you CAN create an attractive and stimulating workout environment on a budget! Some of the items I'm about to list may at first seem silly and perhaps individually not very effective, but together they can make a huge difference in how you experience your treadmill workout. That will have a direct impact on how motivated you may be to hit the treadmill rather than skip it for yet another night.

STIMULATING SIGHTS AND SMELLS

Lighting

Lighting should be both functional and comfortable for working out. I removed one of the lights in my workout area to decrease the lighting so I could more easily view movies or workout videos. If you are watching a computer or video screen and the room is too bright, your eyes will switch back and forth between your laptop screen and the environment lighting causing some irritable eye strain. Conversely, if the room is very dark, your eyes will shift between the treadmill LED panel and the ambient light.

Colours

There is actually much more to colour than meets the eye, so to speak. If your treadmill is in a room with drywall that you can paint, consider the energetic and inviting atmosphere you can create for the price of a can of paint. Of course, colours are associated with various moods, so for a workout room it's important to think about what kind of atmosphere would motivate you to workout.

For example, the colour orange incorporates many of the traits said to be given off by red and yellow to create a vibrant energetic feel. Orange apparently helps with the restoration and balance of our physical energies while providing mental and physical stimulation. I heard about this and figured what the heck, it's worth a try and so I chose 'Orange Zest' (a color made by Behr) to paint one of my larger walls. It also turned out to be a nice compliment beside the cedar wall.

Since workout rooms tend to heat up as the treadmill runs, another interesting choice to consider is a shade of blue. Partly, because blue provides a cooling effect as well as a sense of space. A specific shade known as 'Azure blue' is said to provide inspiration and ambition toward big goals.

If you don't have the time, budget or inclination to paint one or more of your walls, another strategy is to incorporate objects of colour into your workout space to try and achieve similar affects.

Whether you buy into the idea of colours having any kind of impact on your mood or not, it really can't hurt to give it a try. Remember, it's not any one thing you do that will make a huge difference in motivating you to get on the treadmill but every little thing you do collectively.

Mirror, Mirror on the Wall

If possible, put up a good size mirror on the wall adjacent to either side of your treadmill. Mirrors provide the sensation of greater depth and therefore make it look and feel that the room you are in is bigger. For many of you, this can really help to alleviate that sense of being enclosed in an artificial space that feels confined.

Strategically placed mirrors will also provide you with the opportunity to check your posture and overall running

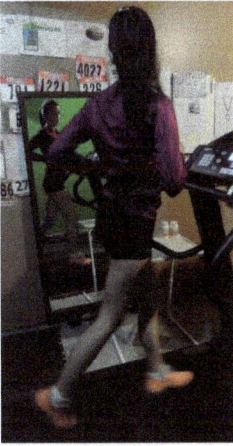

form when you're on the treadmill. As you may know, it's often difficult for us to self-coach when it comes to good running form. We only have our own perception of reality which is not objective. A glance in the mirror will provide you with an unbiased version of what you really look like while you're running. Especially during the later miles of a run when you are beginning to tire and your form starts to suffer.

Just the other day my wife came down to have a quick chat while I was in the final miles of long run and commented that she thought I was leaning forward. That reminded me to have a quick glance sideways in the mirror and I discovered that she was right. When you look sideways, the treadmill frame and console provides some excellent reference points to see what your posture looks like. Are you leaning at the waist, at the neck or nice and straight with a slight lean at the ankles?

I saw a few pictures of myself once during the later stages of a marathon and was shocked to see how horrible my posture was. My head was literally hanging in front of my body. My perception during the run was that I was working hard, felt strong and was running with good posture which was not the case.

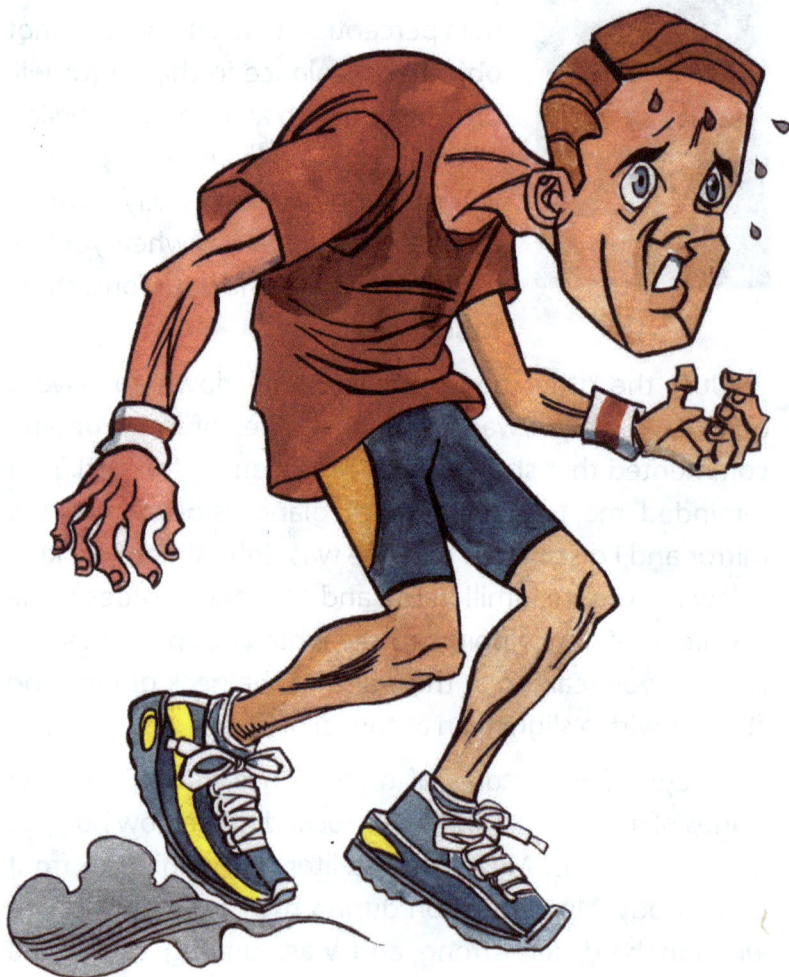

As we discuss in the section on running form, due to the static nature of the treadmill it provides some great opportunities to work on various aspects of your training like your cadence and running form. Inclining the treadmill up to 1% and glancing in a mirror to check yourself periodically throughout your run are two things that can help to correct some bad habits as they occur.

Smells

Heat from the treadmill motor mixed with sweat over time can really produce some nice smells. If you happen to be in an unfinished part of the basement facing cinder blocks, or studs and insulation, do yourself a huge favor and at *least* finish and/or paint the wall that you are facing.

Drywall is a relatively cheap option that you can paint if possible, but you may not be up for the mudding or have a feasible application for drywall.

An interesting alternative to drywall and paint is something I did on a few smaller walls to really enhance the sights and smell of the room I workout in. I installed some thin, rather inexpensive tongue and groove cedar boards in strategic locations on the walls surrounding my treadmill.

Cedar is exceptional for moisture absorption, naturally resists rotting and emits a nice woodsy aroma when it does get wet. You can buy cedar in panels that are designed for closets or as boards and create horizontal or vertical patterns right over existing drywall or to cover up your ugly stud and insulation wall. Most home improvement stores carry a thin variety of cedar boards that work just fine. They are easy to cut, handle and install plus they look (and smell) great!

Using cedar near your treadmill will help absorb some of the moisture (sweat) created over time and emit a really nice outdoor sauna smell.

Marketing people in retail and real estate agents have long known about the powerful potential effects of smell on human behaviour which can be referred to as the Proustian Effect after French author Marcel Proust. He highlighted in his early century novel the connections of smell to memories. Many real estate agents are known to bake up a batch of cookies or a cake as part of their home staging before showing a house to give prospective buyers a sense of well-being and hominess. Other scents such as Jasmine, which encourages relaxation, are used in bedrooms and living rooms.

While you're in the market to take the sweat smell out of your workout room, there is research that demonstrates the fact that **Peppermint Oil** is a powerful motivator to exercise! Aside from stimulating your alertness, peppermint can stimulate your brain in additional ways. The scent travels to the limbic system in your brain, where it affects your hormones and your moods. The smell of peppermint can boost your mood so you feel more refreshed and rejuvenated.

It might also make you crave a candy cane so beware! Experiment to see if this works for you and remember, the motivating effects on the brain are associated to the **smell** of peppermint not the consumption of it.

It can't hurt to try. Should you happen to own a Sentsy unit, they have a few varieties of peppermint that might work well too.

Temperature

You may have heard the sage old running advice to dress as if it will be 20 degrees warmer when running outside. Well, as you may well know, things can really heat up when you're running indoors too. You can increase your duration and enjoyment of the treadmill by employing a few of the following simple cooling methods.

You can keep these close at hand while running:

- Liquids and supplements
- Towels – 1 fresh moist hand towel and 1 to 3 dry
- Fans for cooling (2 or more if possible)

DEREK LALONDE

OTHER MOTIVATORS

Variety – By variety, I mean to vary the training intensity. This technique is both physically as well as mentally important. Running slow all the time trains you to run slow. Intervals, hills, and pacing runs are all exhilarating work outs that improve your speed, stimulate your body to burn fat and keep things exciting. Wherever possible change up your routine including terrain, intensity and running duration. This helps to distribute and vary all of the healthy, yet stressful, impacts on your body. It can also be easier to stay motivated during your training program if you're introducing new sights and sounds to experience during your runs (which may require you to get outside now and again).

Fresh Gear – Whether you're motivated out of guilt because of the amount of money you just spent on your new shoes, or because they feel great compared to your last pair, updating some of your gear can be a great motivation technique to help you look forward to your runs in comfort. As I write this, I sport a very nasty friction burn from using my old running tights 1 long run too many forcing me to take time off and walk funny for a few days. Some lessons are only learned the hard way.

Keeping Track – Keeping track of what you've accomplished, like ticking off a to-do list item, can be very motivating. By writing down the type, intensity and duration of your work outs, you are also building a valuable library of information that you can refer back to if you want to evaluate what training strategies worked well for you.

Inspiring stories and articles – Reading about the training strategies, follies and even physical challenges overcome by other runners can be very motivating. You can also pick up different training tips and tricks to try to keep things fresh as you work toward your goals.

Motivational postings – The motivational sayings or quotes vary by person, but choose what speaks to you and motivates you. Post these in an obvious place in your workout room. Some basic types of sayings include:

Life is short – your life should have purpose

Chasing goals means growth and positive change

Staying focussed on your goal(s) is important to you

A great location would be somewhere that you can easily observe the word(s) while you're running. We can always find excuses, including what might seem like a more ideal time in the future to begin change and start working toward your goals. For this reason, the words that I've found really motivating to me are **Right Now.** I have them printed and located on the same (orange) wall as my immediate goal cards.

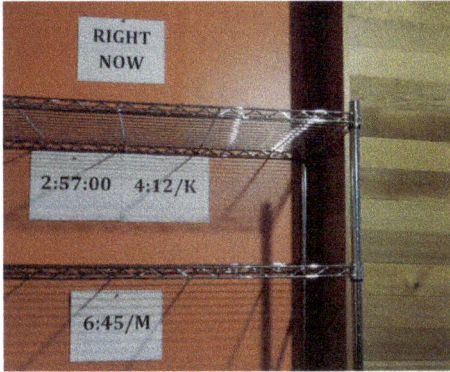

Here are suggestions of some great short motivational words and phrases that you can print and tack up in your workout room. Hopefully at least one or more will resonate with your personality.

MOTIVATING WORDS		MOTIVATING PHRASES
Start	Win	Start Now
Change	Dig	New Body
Live	Breathe	Get Up and Move
Goal	Possible	Your ALL
Discipline	Grow	Go Hard
Try	Action	Don't Quit
Trust	Gain	Born to Run
Better	Run	One Life
Do	Push	One Chance
Focus	Will	One Shot
Today	GO	Right Now
Energy	Engage	It's Go Time
Challenge	Hard	Take Action
Courage	Move	Carpe Diem
Believe	Get	Don't Give up
Commit	Power	Do your BEST
Steady	Best	Never Quit
Strong	Inspire	
Faith		
Hold		
Drive		
Dare		
Risk		

Goal Cards

In addition to motivational words try posting meaningful **numbers** connected to your goals! Specifically, finishing times or running paces that you will be expected to sustain on race day. I like to have a few on the wall directly ahead of my treadmill including the finishing time and average pace of my *immediate goals* which would be something I'm training for that is a few months away.

The key to creating good goal cards is to make sure that you focus on what it is that you do **want** rather than what you don't want. For example, if you want to lose weight you wouldn't put *'STOP EATING'* on the wall but you would capture the exact **weight** that you would like to achieve.

When your mind is connected and focussed on specific numbers, you will be utterly amazed at how in tune your body can get with those numbers; particularly things like running pace. As I've outlined in the heart rate training chapter, this strategy can even work to bring your heart rate down while you're running. Remember, a great goal will have a specific day and time to attached to the distance that you expect to run. When you develop a good race plan, there will be an average pace that you'll need to hold in order to facilitate meeting that goal.

Instructions

1. Establish a crystal clear goal such as the finishing time of a run you are training for.

2. Figure out the average pace that you will need to sustain in order to meet that goal.

3. Using software such as Microsoft Word, create a document with a page layout set to landscape. Select your desired font (I used Cambria) and increase the font size to 175. This size means an entire page will be dedicated to one or to a couple of words at most.

4. Type out your motivating words/times, select them and centre them on the page, and then print.

So a half marathon finishing time of 2 hours will require an average running pace of 9:09 minutes per mile or a 5:41 minutes per km. A full marathon finishing time of 3 hours and 55 minutes will require 8:58.

135 lbs

8:58/mile

Vision Boards

People who use vision boards do not hesitate for a moment to respond when asked "What is it that you really want?"

Vision boards are an awesome way of creating a crystal clear vision of what it is that you want to achieve. It basically involves pasting pictures of the things that you'd like to have and/or achieve onto a board. And, more importantly, they are posted in a place that is in clear view on a daily basis. Vision boards are an excellent way to program your subconscious mind through repetitive exposure.

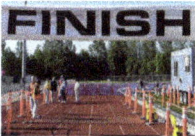

Surround Yourself with Achievements

Probably one of the coolest pieces of memorabilia that I have hanging near my treadmill is dedicated to my first marathon. I ran, and shared, my very first marathon experience with a good friend of mine, John. While it was a painful and interesting day, ultimately we both agreed that it was an extremely rich experience. To capture the moment, John had the great idea of getting our bibs and certificates along with a cool quote mounted within a large picture frame. It is a constant reminder of how hard that first time was and how far I've come since then.

In addition to looking forward and visualizing where you want to go and what you want to achieve, it can help to remind you what you have already accomplished by your hard work. Don't let your race bibs sit in a book or the bottom of your drawer. If you can, post at least a few meaningful ones somewhere near your treadmill. Some, like your first run, may bring you some pride while others might be great reminders of why it is you need to get your butt on the treadmill. Either way, they can be motivating as well as a great way to immerse yourself in your training and racing journey. And that is after all the point, to enjoy the journey.

Learn to Use Focal Points

While training for a 50 km treadmill record, I spent an awful lot of time on the treadmill. Often, during the last miles of my training runs when things were getting tough, I found myself desperately trying to 'zone out', relax and keep a steady pace to endure the leg soreness and overall fatigue.

To help me zone out, I would pick an object about 10 feet straight in front of me to use as a focal point. I also continue to use the same strategy on the treadmill for uncomfortable longer paced runs such as balance point or 'threshold runs'. By 'zone out' I mean getting into a zone of relaxed focus that helps to ignore inner pain while removing outside distractions. Ultra runners must all inevitably find this place in order to find the strength to keep moving forward.

Focussing on a single object helps you to stay in control of your breathing and remove all distractions in the room.

What's really happening, as you are zoning out is that you are connecting your mind and body without obsessing or worrying about how they are working together or what kind of pain you might be experiencing.

Bio-awareness is a sense of awareness of what's going on in your body including your heart rate, sweat rate, energy level, cadence, breathing and it is important. But the trick is to become calmly aware of these signals and respond in like fashion. Take a sip of fuel, wipe your face, relax your breathing, and check your form.

Until you give it a shot, this may sound quite bizarre to you. However, a quick and easy focal point that I've used for years while on the treadmill is a CD that I've hung on the wall underneath my goal card. The vast array of colours created when light rays bounce off of the surface of the disc create a mesmerizing and highly effective focal point.

The best part is this is cheap and easy to do. Grab any old CD you have laying around that you don't use any more. Place a thumbtack on the wall and place the hole of the CD over it at eye level directly in front of your treadmill or somewhere easy for you to see while running.

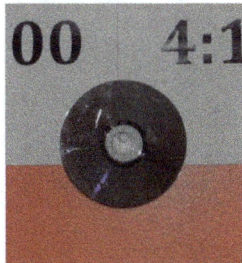

DEREK LALONDE

•C•

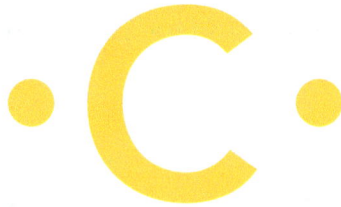

ENGAGE IN STIMULATING ACTIVITIES

Music

Little compares to your favourite music to get you moving and having fun while running. If you are willing to take the time to construct a playlist of your favourite tunes, try and give some consideration to the placement of the songs relative to the energy level required. For example, typical songs are 3 to 5 minutes in length so place songs in your list that you enjoy but don't necessarily make you feel like going hard until after a good warm up period of 15 to 20 minutes.

Another consideration when constructing your running playlist, is having songs with a tempo of at least **180** steps per minute. There is ample research that suggests a cadence of this rate co-relates with good running form. **Treadflix.com** has CD compilations of **'Blacklungz'** music that was created for the running videos and all of the music falls between 90 and 95 bpm. Keep this in mind if you acquire the videos and happen to enjoy the music on the videos!

Movies

Watching a movie is one of the greatest ways to pass the time while you're on the treadmill; particularly if you are a distance runner and logging 2 to 5 hour runs. A great way to motivate yourself to get on the treadmill any given week night is to have a rule that you can only watch your favourite episodes of a series on the treadmill. This has worked brilliantly for me over the years. In fact, it may have worked too well. I almost ran myself into the ground when I got hooked on 'Breaking Bad' and couldn't wait to see each next episode.

TREADFLIX

It was a burning desire to create stimulating, effective training visualization tools that would help occupy my time on the treadmill that led to the creation of the first TREADFLIX movie. And of course what's a video without music? I collaborated with a good friend, who happens to be a great musician and was eager to take on the challenge of creating music that would suit runners. As we worked together, the treadmill training videos slowly came to fruition.

TREADFLIX

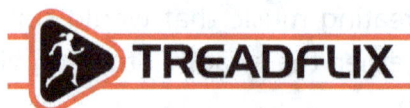

Marathon Series

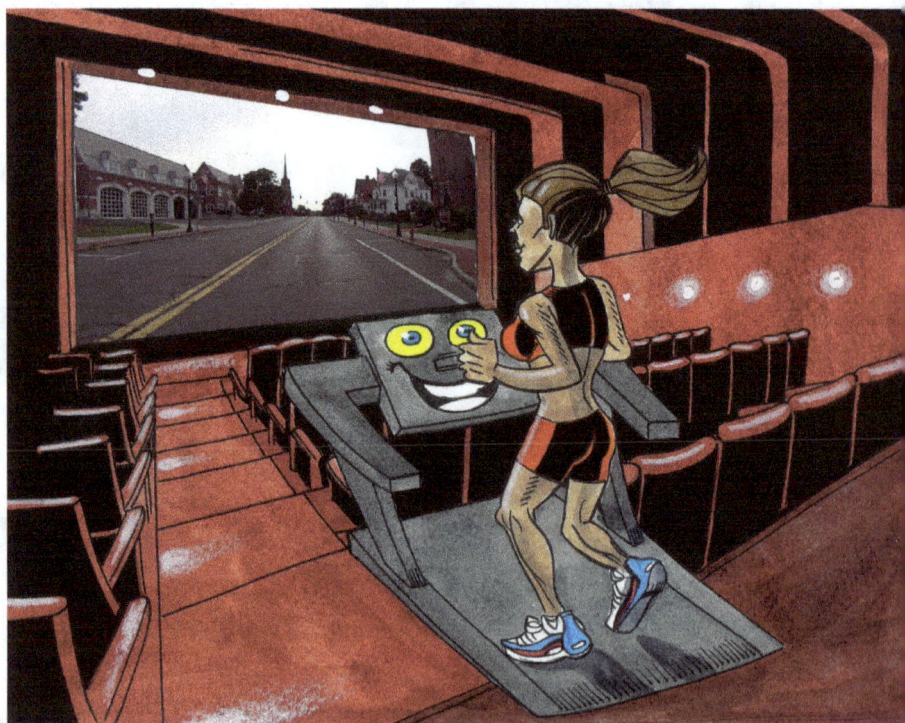

RUN BOSTON!

At **TREADFLIX.COM** there are, as of now, **3** courses available for purchase (and many more in development) including the **3** North American major marathons **Boston, New York and Chicago!**

Each course provides a 1 hour and 2 hour workout option so they're unbeatable if you are looking to do a quick daily workout or want to do fun and relevant training on the treadmill for the duration of a longer run.

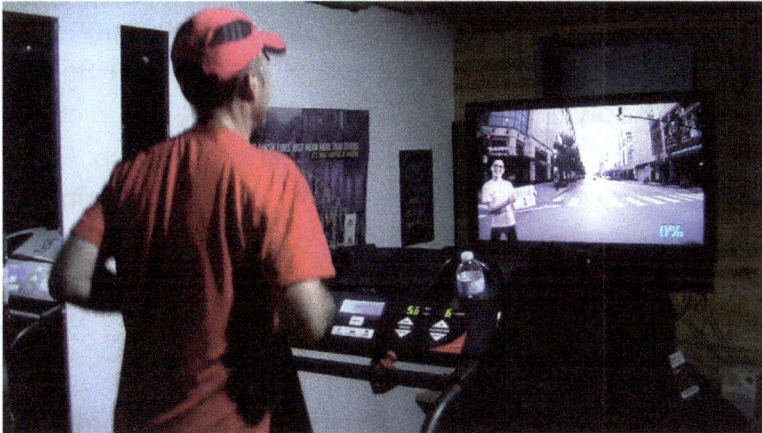

Running Downhill on a Treadmill

It's no big secret, that the best way to get ready for any event that you are training for is to mimic the demands of the actual event while in training. For courses that you have never run and are training for, be on particular lookout for course descriptions that include the terms 'scenic' and 'gently rolling hills' as a clue that your training should include some downhill running.

In fact, unless you are training for a course that is 'pancake flat', you'll come up a little short on race day without any kind of training on a decline. The reason for this physiologically, is that downhill running places unique and specific demands on your quad muscles and the ligaments supporting your knees. Even with excellent running form and letting yourself go, running on a decline causes a braking motion that your legs achieve through concentric muscle contractions.

Many first time runners of the Boston marathon learn the value of incorporating some downhill running into training the hard way. Since the first 4 miles of Boston are on a downhill grade, these concentric contractions are squeezed from the quads very early in the run. Much later through miles 21 to 23, many well trained runners are shocked to find their legs 'cooked' without good explanation.

Climbing hills are easy enough to simulate on the treadmill. However, what goes up usually comes down as well. So as the #1 fan of training on a treadmill for events of ANY distance, I'm here to say that the lack of decline running is without a doubt the treadmill's biggest deficiency as a training tool – but it doesn't have to be! While most treadmills don't offer a decline option (few do) there is a **very cheap and simple solution** to this short coming of an otherwise awesome sport-specific running tool.

A Short Story of Discovery

After using a level and measuring tape to evaluate the inclines on my treadmill, I discovered that each degree of incline equates to approximately ½ inch. In other words, a 3% incline raises the front of the treadmill 1 and ½ inches from when it was level. The great news is this height equates perfectly to the typical height of a 2" piece of lumber. The other great news is, these measurements are virtually the same for any treadmill regardless of make and model.

In my application, since my deck is 30" wide, I used a 32" length of 2" x 6" pine board to place under the back feet of my treadmill to simulate a downgrade. I used a 2 x 6 to ensure that I had plenty of room for the back feet of the treadmill as I wanted to minimize the possibility of the feet sliding off. I have had this piece of wood in place for close to 2 years now.

Now, when I put the treadmill to 3%, my treadmill is perfectly level which of course equates to your treadmill being at 0% incline. Since I always run with a 1% incline, this now means my treadmill is regularly set to 4%.

Of course, when the treadmill is at 0%, this raising of the rear feet creates the equivalent downhill grade of about **-3%**. While there are certainly steeper downhill grades out in the real world, even the smallest setting of 2% (which is now the equivalent of -1%), is enough to invoke those muscle contractions.

At first, I was sceptical about the value of going through the trouble of having a -3% decline on my treadmill. This scepticism very quickly vanished the first day after running at the smallest decline (2%) for only 15 minutes at the end of a run. I was surprised at the amount of quad soreness that I had the following few days. This really opened my eyes to the importance of working some decline running into treadmill training. Since then, that 2 x 6 board has remained snugly tucked under the rear of my treadmill and I've incorporated at least a few bouts of decline running into my weekly routine.

Please keep in mind, that like runners, not all treadmills are alike! While I've personally had many years of flawless operation with my treadmill propped up at the back with a piece of wood, you should find out if YOUR treadmill can handle the extra stress created by the change in position. My treadmill has a hefty 4 HP motor and so you may want to consult with your treadmill manufacturer if you have any doubts about yours!

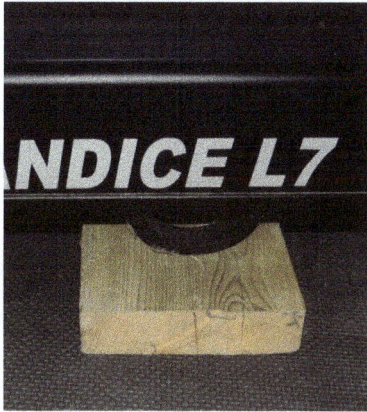

Instructions:

1. Measure the width of your treadmill deck. This length plus 2 extra inches is the length of 2 x 6 that you will need to place under the feet.

2. For maximum safety, centre the feet in the middle of the wood with an equal amount of overlap on either side. Also, to avoid movement of the wood and treadmill, your treadmill should be on a proper rubber exercise mat or foam flooring.

3. With the rear block in place, your new 0 is now 3% incline. If you are using the '1% is zero' rule with your treadmill then of course an incline of 4% will be your default setting to start your runs at.

Safety warning

Just like any hard running workouts, downhill running carries risks - particularly if you've never done it before. As highlighted above, downhill running simulates a muscular 'braking' motion known as a concentric muscle contraction during your ground contact phase. This response can make mincemeat of your quads and place extra stress on your knees.

So, be sure to adequately warm up, keep your first downhill workouts to very short bouts of 5 minutes at 1% decline until you can safely adjust to the new stresses of the decline. Each week, **slowly** incorporate more time or decline as you become stronger and your body learns how to protect you through this running dynamic.

Keep in mind also that downhill workouts are probably just *not worth the risk* if you are not training for an event with little to no significant declines.

Design Your Running Theatre on a Budget

The following setup is a great way to quickly and easily have your audio and visuals for treadmill running without compromising good running posture. When the treadmills with built-in screens first came out I thought that was such a great idea. I quickly discovered however, by trying a few in the gym and at the store, that looking at the built-in screen that close caused a bit of dizziness. This makes some sense, because when you are running your head is bobbing slightly up and down. Even runners with excellent form experience some vertical body movement while running.

Running at home, with my laptop perched on top of a tray close to the machine, I experienced similar dizziness and so I was really disappointed. I never had a problem watching the TV, however, which was situated about 15 feet away. The issue was that I really wanted to use my laptop which was portable, and easily accommodates being able to watch movies on Netflix , the TREADFLIX marathon videos and my favourite downloaded TV episodes. The challenge was not only having the laptop the right distance from me but also at the right height so that I could comfortably see it above the console while maintaining good upright posture while I ran.

One fateful day I happened to notice a painting ladder leaning in the corner. I set it up about 3 feet in front of the treadmill and placed the laptop on the top step of the ladder. I then noticed that the paint can tray which flips out had a perfect amount of room for my laptop speakers which I promptly put into place and voila! I found both the distance and height perfect to maintain posture while eliminating dizziness.

It's also very mobile so if necessary, you can simply fold the ladder and lean it against the wall and out of the way until your next run.

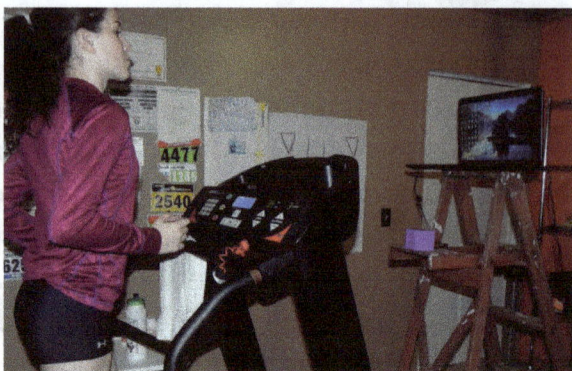

So while I found that the ideal distance for me was 3 feet, you might like it even a bit further and perhaps higher. So it's very likely that you have experienced that same vertigo when trying to watch a movie on a close screen while running. Try the painting ladder setup!

Your spouse *may* object to the painting ladder if your treadmill is in a more common area of the house.

You might also experience a similar dizzy sensation with too little lighting in the room. I'm not a big fan of super bright lights in the room where my treadmill is located mainly because I often watch movies on my laptop. I also just find bright lights annoying, but that's just me. Remember, it's all about creating a setting that is appealing and stimulating to **you**.

If you have all of the lights off, your eyes will constantly adjust between the LED lights on your treadmill panel and the light from the monitor or TV that you are watching ahead of you. This eye movement is not a conscious adjustment that you necessarily notice, but it is enough to contribute to eye strain and vertigo. Not to mention the fact that, some extra lighting while you're on the treadmill makes it safer and easier on your spacial perception so that you don't wander off the belt.

HOW IS YOUR RUNNING FORM?

Before getting into treadmill training, I think it's critical to have a good look at the importance of good running form. When I have spoken to people about working on their running form, I've heard them make comments like "I'm not that serious about running…I only run for fun" or "I'm a beginner so I'm not quite ready for that yet." Well, good running form reduces impact to your body and helps you to run lighter, faster and for a much longer time span in your life. What's not more fun about that? There is no better time than when you are learning to run to adopt the right habits!

I should point out that often, and even in this book, you'll see the phrases 'running form' and 'running technique' used interchangeably. It might help to think of the two terms separately though. Where running form is how your body looks during the different stages of running, running technique would be the actual mechanics or movements you make while running.

There is quite a lot of information and research out

there on what constitutes good running form but not a whole lot specifically focussing on running form while on the treadmill. Much of the same information about good form can, however, be applied whether you are outside or on the treadmill.

Since good running form and technique does not come naturally for most of us, it's something we need to practice repeatedly, like a golf swing, until it becomes more instinctive or natural feeling. Even then, it's important to check your form on a regular basis to see where you're at, particularly during the later stages of longer runs and races.

Checking your Form

One way to have your form analyzed is by setting up a video camera with a tripod at a local track. You can leave it running for the duration of your run and capture yourself every few minutes as you pass in front of the camera. At **www.treadflix.com** I have a brief video regarding running form on a treadmill that you might find helpful.

Of course, the same setup while running on the treadmill will yield you much more continuous running footage that you can watch later. You simply place the video camera recording device directly beside you far enough away to get your whole body in the picture. Treadmill running also makes it easy to have a peek at your form via a mirror on the wall on either side of the machine.

So, once you're able to see what you look like while running, here are some of the basic elements of good form that you can compare yourself to:

- **Good posture** with head over torso, chest slightly puffed out

- **Relaxed shoulders**, arms slightly bent and wrists along sides of the body

- **Slight body lean** forward from the ankles, not from the waist*

- **Feet are under body as they touch ground**

*The only significant difference to speak of in your running form when you're running on the treadmill versus outside is your body lean. Since the belt is simulating your forward momentum there is no need to lean and fall forward from the ankles as you would on solid ground.

Since you probably don't exclusively run on the treadmill and do train for events that will be run outside, it's important to simulate the lean so that you are as close to the same running form as possible. Setting the treadmill to a 1% grade allows you to run upright with good posture while accomplishing a slight lean.

Minimize Running Impact

If you could care less about the physics of running and just want to know the bottom line, hop down to '**The Bottom Line'** section a little later in this book. Otherwise, please keep reading.

The main difference between running on the treadmill and running over ground occurs when your feet touch the surface you are running on, which is known as the 'ground contact phase'.

When running over the ground, you are falling slightly forward and catching yourself. As each foot touches the ground it supports and balances your body weight momentarily before switching off support to the opposite foot coming in for a landing to take over the task.

On a treadmill, when your supporting foot comes into contact with the moving belt, it pulls your foot backward. From a muscle coordination perspective, preventing your feet and body from being pulled backward is a different scenario than preventing yourself from falling forward.

The belt is in motion during ground contact and is one of the contributors to the treadmill having better shock absorption.

However as you'll see, treadmills actually help to promote good running form by teaching you to lift your feet quicker than you would otherwise need to outside.

Now, let's have a look at the impacts of running on your body to highlight the importance and objective of good running form. While there are technical differences between running on a treadmill versus running over ground, in both cases your body is being supported temporarily by the foot that is touching the surface you are running on.

As soon as your foot makes contact, the impact from your weight is being transferred onto that surface. The following variables determine how much impact is generated and what path the impact shockwave will take as the energy is dissipated:

- The density of the running surface
- Angle and point of contact by legs/feet
- Speed of feet coming down for contact/support

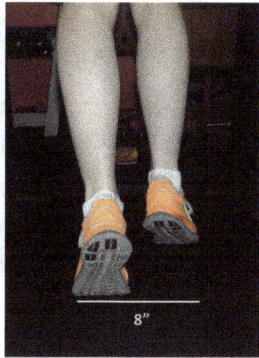

Technique - Training your Body to Run Softly

If you focus on one thing, many other components of good running form will follow including:

- Quick cadence
- Landing more toward the balls of your feet
- Having your feet directly under your body
- Letting your feet fall naturally back down

That one thing is **minimizing your ground contact time**. In other words, practice getting your feet off the ground as soon as they touch.

A really great way to train your body and brain is to **run barefoot** on your treadmill. Socks are actually a good idea to minimize any kind of friction burns on your feet from the belt. Of course you can opt to run barefoot outside as well, however for safety and impact, choose your surface wisely such as a groomed golf course or soccer/football field.

Running barefoot allows all of the nerves along the bottoms of your feet to be engaged in the ground contact phase while you run. As you can imagine, your feet will naturally not want to experience abrupt high impact nor will your body want your heels to strike the ground first. Think of a time where you've perhaps crossed a hot paved driveway or road barefoot. Your natural tendency will be to get up off your heels. For these two reasons doing some of your training in bare feet really helps to promote great running form with low impact.

The Bottom Line

Treadmills are excellent training tools to aid in developing good running technique while minimizing impact on your body. And this is great news because learning to run 'softly' is one of the keys to a healthy long term running career. Soft running means running in such a way that minimizes the impact on your body when your feet hit the ground.

While treadmills do have far superior shock absorbing capabilities versus most outdoor terrain; it's still very important to run with good technique on the treadmill in order to take full advantage of this benefit. It's still possible to get injured on a treadmill by running with bad form.

Running cadence is a very close relative of good running form since quick turnover means as little ground contact as possible. Running cadence, also known as a runner's rhythm, can be quite simply defined as the turnover rate of the feet or legs. It is commonly expressed as revolutions per minute in either total or single steps. The understanding and, more importantly, the application of proper running cadence, is critical to employing correct running form. There is very strong evidence, from data gathered through analysis of elite runners with excellent technique and running economy, that the ideal cadence is a minimum of 180 steps per minute(SPM), or **90 SPM for each foot**. Surprisingly, cadence does not seem to vary more than a couple of single steps per minute when comparing drastically different paces for any individual runner.

For many years, I have been in the habit of counting (secretly) the cadence of runners from all levels. One thing that I have concluded from my observations that prove true time and time again is that runners with poor running form have a cadence that is either slightly below, or well below, 180 foot-steps per minute (SPM). The explanation for this that seems to jump out is that all of the elements of bad running form - such as over-striding with resulting heel striking - make it very difficult to maintain a brisk cadence. This is why I believe one of the first things you should do to help your running form is to first become of aware of what your cadence is, and then continually work at improving it.

Check Your Cadence

An easy way to measure your running cadence , is to count how many times your right foot hits the ground in any given minute. You can do this anywhere if you have a watch or are on a treadmill. Once you have your number, work at squeezing one or more extra steps in the next minute. Follow this with relaxing back to what felt like your normal cadence. This little drill is also known as 'quick feet' and this helps to improve your rate of hamstring muscle firing which is the fundamental component of brisk cadence. Not only is this a great exercise to help improve your running form, but it helps to pass the time on those lonely longer runs. It can be fun to see how many steps you can squeeze into a minute.

When you employ correct running form , you are working in harmony with nature and therefore with the laws of gravity. For this reason, an increase in your running pace should translate to an increase in running cadence or otherwise known as leg turnover. Think about the actions of the wheel of a bicycle. As the bike moves forward, the wheel turns. The number of times the wheel makes a full revolution in any given minute increases as the speed of the bicycle increases. In a perfect world, so too would a runners cadence but you have to train your brain and muscles so that they can fire as rapidly as you need them to.

Quick Feet for Running Form

You might think that training to hit the ground more frequently would actually increase the pounding to your body however just the opposite is true. When you increase the number of times your feet hit the ground a few changes occur in your running form.

To accommodate the quicker cadence, your hamstrings fire quicker, your heels come up faster and as a result your stride shortens since you simply don't have time to make those huge strides that would otherwise drive your feet out in front of your body.

So the main benefit of a shorter stride is helping you to move away from landing on your heels, or 'heel striking'- the true culprit to unnecessary running impact and the 'arch' enemy of running speed! Runners of any level can practice increasing their running cadence because cadence is not pace related. It is just as easy to lift your heels straight up under your butt at 180 steps per minute going 5 miles/hour as it is at 9 miles/hour. The difference is 180 *or more* steps per minute come more naturally when you are running fast.

So let's look once again at the elements of good technique, and what you should look like while executing it:

- Good posture from head to toe
- Relaxed shoulders
- Wrists brushing along the sides of the hips
- Body falling forward at the ankles
- Feet coming quickly straight up under the body
- Feet falling naturally back down
- Brisk cadence

Running Technique Drills

Running drills that will allow you to practice good running technique include the following:

Quick feet – this drill really works on your hamstring muscle firing and helps to move toward a faster cadence.

Instructions:

Without changing your pace or incline, see how many times you can tap your feet on the belt in any given minute. Focus on bringing your feet straight up under your body as soon as they touch the belt. Let your feet fall down rather than drive them down for each contact. Shoot for 100 single steps per minute! After each minute take a minute or two of your regular comfortable cadence for recovery.

Falling Lunge – this helps teach your body the sensation of working with gravity by falling forward from the ankles while running.

Instructions:

With good posture, let your body **fall** forward from the ankles. At the last possible moment, extend one leg to catch yourself ending in a lunge position.

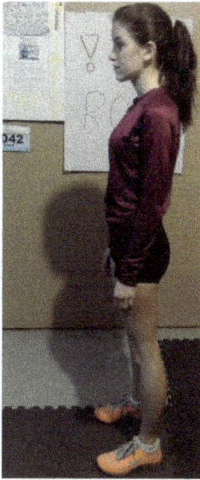

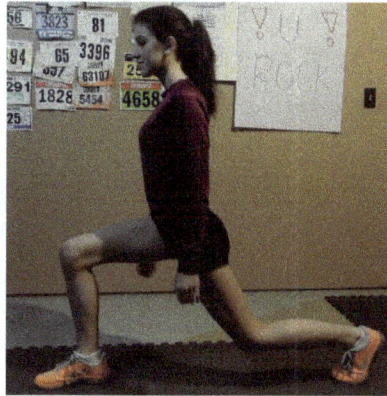

Single Leg Hops – this drill helps to teach the sensation of bringing your feet up as soon as they touch the ground.

Instructions:

Starting in a standing position or on the treadmill with the treadmill off, perform mini hops. Every second or third hop, lift one foot straight up under your butt, and let it fall straight back down. Perform 5 to 10 hops then continue hopping and lifting one leg while moving forward.

After working one leg for a definite period of time, repeat for the other leg.

TIP: A fun and effective way to apply the quick feet running drills, is through the use of good running music. Good running music should range between **90 to 98 BPM** which, if you run along to and keep the beat, trains your body to produce a quick turnover in a fun and motivating way!

Keep in mind that **all TREADFLIX videos** also contain running music that was intentionally created at the **90 to 96 bpm range**. A band known as **'Blacklungz'** was commissioned to create all of the music for the treadmill videos. Their (downloadable) CD of just running music called **Second Wind** can be purchased at **TREADFLIX. com**.

BUILD YOUR OWN TRAINING PROGRAM

Many treadmills have pre-programmed workouts that you can take advantage of but you should be familiar with what each program entails. Training smart means that you **know the exact training purpose** of every workout to avoid injury and make the most of your training time. For example, you would not want to necessarily repeat the same program day after day or week after week.

The various workouts below differ in length, simulated terrain and intensity so collectively they properly prepare you for your running goals by causing specific physiological adaptations. Each workout includes a brief description, training purpose and instructions for proper execution so that you have full control over the run.

I have categorized all of the workouts into different 'buckets' to make them clear to understand from an intensity/effort point of view. The best way to make the most out of your time and to keep yourself in adaptation and recovery mode is to constantly vary all of the workouts in any given week.

*If you don't have the time to build your own training program, I have a wide variety of free downloadable and printable training programs available at:

www.meet-your-running-goals.com/running-training-program.html

EASY	MEDIUM	HARD
Cross Train	Aerobic Run	Speed work
Walk	Drills	Long Run
Rest Day	Medium Long Run	Temp/Pace Run
Easy Run		

TRAINING PROGRAM

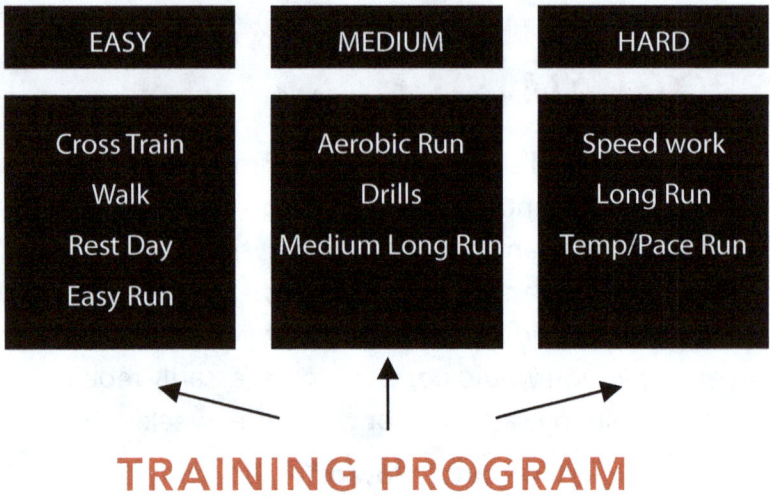

At the end of the process, a training week should ideally look something like this:

Monday	Tuesday	Wednesday	Thursday	Friday	Saturday	Sunday
Easy	Medium	Hard	Easy	Medium	Hard	Easy

Therefore there is only **one golden rule** when using the bucket system to build your own training program - **You must pick from each bucket once before picking a second time from any bucket.**

For example, if you start building your program on a Monday, Monday through Wednesday must have a workout from each bucket. On Thursday you can start the process over… one from each bucket. It is recommended, but not always essential, that each hard workout is followed by an easy workout.

This really depends on your experience level, specific goals and individual physiology. There will be times in a program where a runner intends to do strategic back to back long runs on Saturday and Sunday as part of an endurance training program. However, I will put out there, that **ALL** runners need recovery time built in to their program regardless of level to ensure progress, and avoid injury and/or burnout.

Dynamite results require dynamic training!

TREADMILL WORKOUTS

Whether you are running outside, solely on a treadmill or a combination of both, a wide variety of running workouts make up a well-balanced running training program! Since the purpose of this book is to learn many ways that you can leverage the awesomeness of your treadmill's ability to help you train, each workout has been specifically customized to be performed on the treadmill.

HILLS (SPEED AND STRENGTH)

Workout purpose

They simultaneously build muscular, cardiovascular and respiratory strength – not to mention a solid dose of mental toughness (every runner's best friend). Hills are also like sport specific weight training for runners. Every well-balanced training program should have some type of hill workout at least every couple of weeks.

Some of the workouts described below include a **downhill** component which of course is completely optional. However, recognize that if you are training for a hilly course on a treadmill without making the downhill adjustment, you will be partially underprepared for this demand on race day.

Often we train really well for a course and are surprised at how sore our quads are afterwards. Yes, running intensity during a race differs than that of most training runs, but it is the rigors of going downhill that I believe we underestimate and therefore are underprepared for. Especially if most, or all, of your training occurs on a treadmill or flat running route.

One final statement about decline running on your treadmill; **Be sure to thoroughly warm up, and then integrate these workouts very gradually into your program. Keep your downhill intervals well under 5 minutes.**

Hill Tips

It's virtually impossible to overextend and strike the ground hard with your heels when running up an incline, which is why hill training is good for practicing proper running form. When running up hills it's important to focus on good posture rather than leaning into the hill by bending at the waist. Your head should be up high and shoulders relaxed.

Before running hills consider doing some ballistic stretching after your warm up miles targeting your calves, hamstrings and lower back.

1. Hill repeats

If you do these bi-weekly, they will really help to carve the serious athlete that lies within you. Hill repeats can, and should be, varied each time you do them both in duration and steepness.

Instructions:

- Warm up with little to no incline for 1.5 to 2 miles.
- If desired, hop off treadmill and perform some ballistic stretching.
- At a steady, but still aerobic pace, kick your incline up to the desired level. 3% is mild and 10% is aggressively steep.
- Hold for a set amount of time – 1 minute for really steep and up to 5 minutes for a small incline.
- Bring treadmill back down to your base incline and recover for a couple of minutes before kicking the incline up again.
- Continue to repeat the process of running inclines followed by recovery periods.

2. 'Kili'

Named after Africa's Mount Kilimanjaro, this is a very gentle and gradual mountain climb at a moderate incline. Slow and steady gets you there in one piece.

Instructions:

- After 1.5 to 2 mile warm up put the treadmill to **3% incline** (**6** if your treadmill is raised with a 2′″ x 6″ in the back).

- Add 1% every **5 to 10 minutes** depending on the total time of your workout.

- Maintain the same starting speed throughout the entire run.

- With **5 minutes left**, bring treadmill down to starting incline as a cool down.

3. Everest

Some courses just have a nasty steep hill or two which take a big piece out of many runners. If you can get good at running hills like this, you'll fare much better on the other side and return quicker to your controlled breathing. Of course, you can walk this one too and still get a great workout in.

Instructions:

- After 1.5 to 2 mile warm up at your level/starting incline at an easy pace, raise the treadmill incline by 6% to 9%.

- **Hang on** for a minimum of ¼ mile (400 m) repeats or the equivalent of between **2-4 minutes** before bringing the incline back to original level setting (0% or 1%).

- Repeat the process of incline followed by a recovery until the end of the workout.

4. Gently Rolling Course

Every time I see these words contained within a running course description (typically in a marketing brochure), I have to laugh. The words 'gently' and 'rolling' to give the sense of something fun and wavy. It's usually a positive spin on a hilly course so be ready to bring your lungs! In any case, now you know, and this workout will help prepare you for this type of course. These basically differ from the previous hill workouts in that each incline interval is followed by a *decline* interval prior to going back to level recovery running. Adding the decline option more realistically simulates a gently rolling course. After all, what goes up must come down…right?

Instructions:

- After 1.5 to 2 mile warm up at your level/starting incline at an easy pace, raise the treadmill incline by **3% to 5%.**

- After **2 minutes**, bring the incline down to **-2%** and hold for 2 more minutes.

- Follow this up and down interval with 2 minutes of level running before repeating the process until the end of your run.

5. Walk the Plank
- Incline to Exhaustion

Instructions:

- After 1.5 to 2 mile warm up at your level/starting incline at an easy pace, raise the treadmill incline by 1**%.**

- Continue to raise the incline by 1% **every ¼ mile until exhaustion.**

- It might be a good idea to hop on the sides of the treadmill while dropping your incline back down to 0% when you're done.

- Walk off at least ½ mile cool down.

6. The Switch

This is a great combo workout that provides hill and leg turnover work. While it's challenging it's interesting mentally as well as physically since the training focus switches half way through the run. The first half focuses on building a steady incline to a peak followed by a switch to less incline and more speed to the end. This workout should be about 60 minutes in length.

Instructions:

- Start the treadmill at **1%** incline and a very easy warm up pace.

- After 10 minutes, increase the incline by **2%.**

- Continue to increase by **2%** every **5** minutes until **30** minutes.

- At 30 minutes, drop incline by **2%** and increase your speed by **1 mph.**

- Continue to drop incline by **2%** and increase pace by **1 mph** every **5** minutes until you've reached **60 minute** mark.

- Cool down with your easy starting pace.

SPEED-WORK

While your pace and running cadence are closely linked, there are many other bodily systems at play that become taxed as you increase running speed. Therefore, it's important to note that the ability to increase and/or sustain any given pace not only depends on increasing your cadence, but also depends on the synergy of:

1. **Muscle firing/contraction capabilities (hamstrings)**

2. **Respiration rate**

3. **Energy conversion capabilities (Aerobic – presence of oxygen and, at quicker paces, anaerobic capacity – lactate utilization/buffering & maximum oxygen uptake/VO2max)**

4. **Mental capacity to sustain pace**

Depending on a runner's goals (distance, speed), each factor can be simulated through various types of speed work training to be more effective and lead to an increased ability to achieve and hold a given pace. This training effect will invariably improve the runner's economy so less effort is required to achieve the running pace than before.

There are some good reasons for incorporating various types of speedwork into your training. One obvious benefit is you will be able to run and complete your goals faster. Also, periodic intervals of running at a faster pace are more stressful on many of your body systems and therefore invoke a training response making you stronger and faster. Specifically, your heart which is at the center of your operations, becomes larger stronger and more efficient at pumping oxygen rich blood to your working muscles.

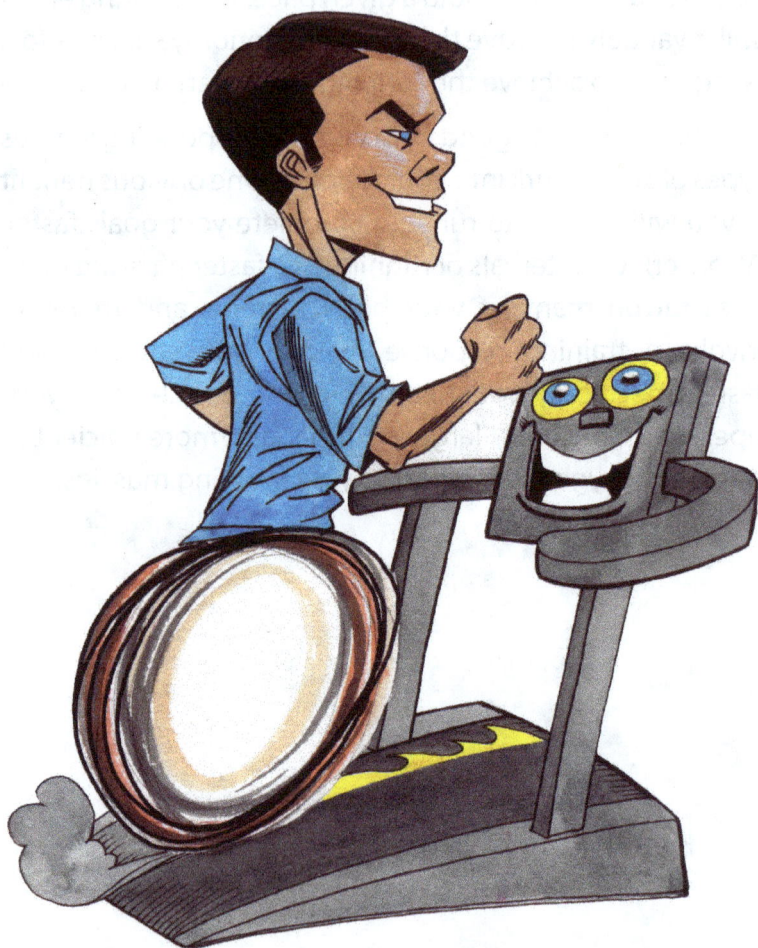

Why Care about Running Faster?

There is a very simple answer to this. Running fast is invigorating and fun and is an excellent fat burning stimulus for your body. As a bonus, you will also become a more efficient runner overall across the spectrum of paces.

Speed includes intervals workouts, which are most commonly done on an outdoor track, and have a wide range of frequency, distances and intensities which depend on the specific event that a runner is preparing for.

One final note about speed work – ample warm up in addition to some ballistic stretching which can be in the form of some easy running, is a very good idea. Running fast pushes the limits of your body systems and to avoid injury you want to make sure that these systems are warm and ready for action. The best way to do this is to warm up for a good mile of easy running, followed by some ballistic (moving) stretching off the treadmill before tackling your workout.

1. Intervals

These are your run of the mill track workouts that you simply perform on the treadmill. Intervals are periods of sustained speed followed by a brief recovery period. Most treadmills, even those dating back 15 years, have basic interval programs on them. You might want to have a look at what you have to see if it may meet your needs and save you from having to touch buttons at a blistering pace.

There is a real excitement in going super-fast on a treadmill. In particular, I think often you are forced to dig a little deeper during your final intervals just to maintain the speed of the belt when you might tend to fade on a real track. Of course, if you fade on the treadmill you're going flying off the belt which is even more motivation!

Interval workouts generally range from 100 to 1600 meters in length. If you're 5k training you might focus more on shorter faster intervals of 100 to 800 meters in length. Longer, slightly slower intervals of 800 to 1600 meters in length yield more of a benefit if you're training for a half and full marathon.

Instructions:

- After 1 to 1.5 mile warm up (and ballistic stretching if desired) enter the desired pace of your run e.g. 8.6 mph.

- Run the length of your interval e.g. 800m = 0.5 mile.

- Bring the speed down to a walking pace for the duration of your recovery. Recovery should last approximately **half of the distance** of your interval. So an 800 meter repeat would be followed by a brisk 400 m walk/easy run. Recovery is an individual choice however it should be long enough for your heart rate to fall well into the **lower end of your aerobic zone**.

- Repeat the above process for the desired number

of repetitions. A high quality session will have between 2 and 4 miles worth of total speed distance.

2. Stairway to Heaven (a.k.a. Speed Ladder)

This is a great overall speed workout that involves a gradual build-up of pace. It's best done on a flat incline. The objective is to go as fast as you can possibly go, without flying off the treadmill, until exhaustion. Executed correctly, being finished should feel like 'heaven'.

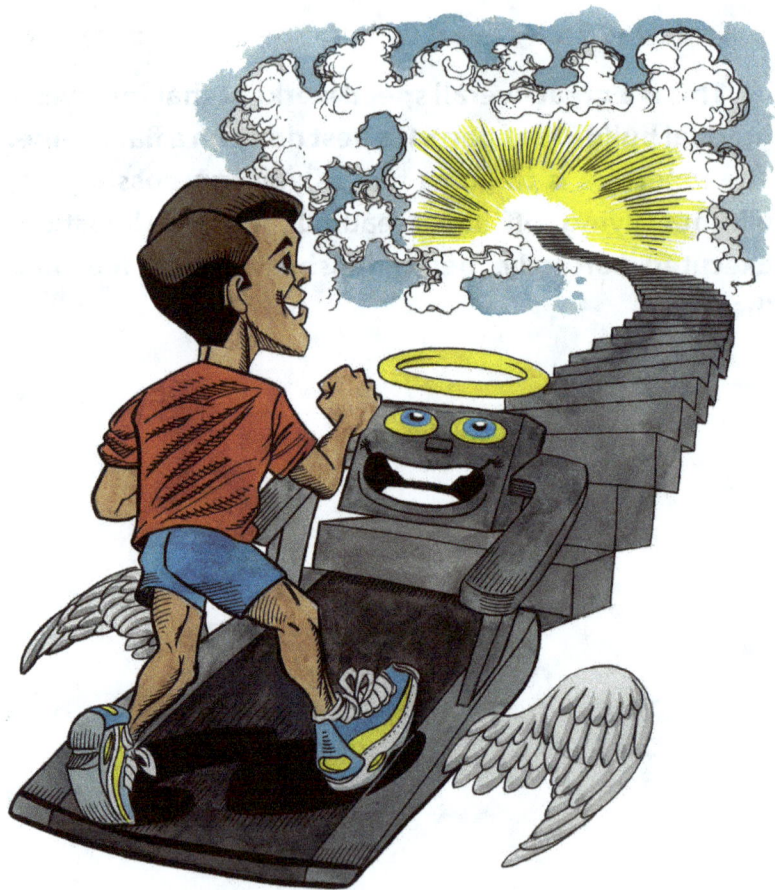

Instructions:

- After 1.5 to 2 mile warm up at your level incline at an **easy pace**, increase the pace by **0.5 mph.**

- Continue to raise the pace by **0.5 mph every ½ mile until exhaustion.**

- Bring pace back down to warm up pace and run for ¼ mile until finally cooling down for at least another ½ mile.

3. Lactate Balance Point (LBP) runs a.k.a. Tempo or Threshold runs

To be performed correctly, these are running workouts that require a good awareness (preferably through lactate blood analysis) of your training zone known as the lactate balance zone. The unscientific way to describe the pace for this zone is the pace that you can hold if you ran as fast as you could without fading for approximately 1 hour to 1 hour and 15 minutes. For many runners this is close to their fastest half marathon pace. Another crude way to describe this pace is just below the pace where you would be 'huffing and puffing'.

Any way you slice it LBP runs are workouts that I have always loved to hate. They are particularly uncomfortable and require great focus to keep your heart rate in control. They do however teach a runner's brain and body to sustain aggressive speeds for prolonged periods of time. This workout is an excellent training stimulus for more advanced half and full marathoners looking for a breakthrough performance.

Just as long runs teach your body how to spare muscle glycogen and use stored body fat for fuel, LBP runs teach your body how to become good at converting energy aerobically close to, or at, your anaerobic zone by spending time just below, or at, the bottom of this zone. As a result, the zone occurs later or at a higher heart rate and pace.

There are two ways to execute these runs which I've outlined below. I'm a bigger believer in *Option 1*, which I also think is harder, because I feel that it more closely mimics real conditions where opportunities for recovery periods do not present themselves.

Option 1 – Continuous Tempo Run
Instructions:

- For tempo runs it's beneficial to warm up for at least 2 and up to 4 miles with the first 15 minutes being at an easy pace, followed by a gradual climb in speed.

- These runs can be done at level or an optional 1% and up to 2% grade. An increase in grade will be more difficult and so you'll require less speed to get to the right heart rate.

- Increase the speed to your desired level and hold that pace for a minimum of 20 minutes. Work your way up gradually over several weeks to spending

45 minutes at that pace. If you're training by heart rate (you smart devil) don't be shy to adjust the pace if you start to experience some cardiac drift above your acceptable zone.

- Decrease the treadmill speed to a slow run and/or brisk walk to cool down for at least 10 minutes.

Option 2 – Tempo Intervals

Instructions:

- For tempo runs it's beneficial to warm up for at least 2 and up to 4 miles with the first 15 minutes being at an easy pace, followed by a gradual climb in speed.

- These runs can be done at level or an optional 1% and up to 2% grade. An increase in grade will be more difficult and so require less speed to get to the right heart rate.

- Increase the speed to your desired level and hold that pace for 1 mile.

- Decrease the speed to a slow run/brisk walk for 3 minutes.

- Resume the previous pace and continue to run/ take a break for 4 to 7 miles.

- Once your last interval is complete, do a slow run and/or brisk walk to cool down for at least 10 minutes.

Option 3 - Middle Cut Down Tempo

This is a beautifully difficult workout given to me by the great ultra-marathon legend **Paul DeWitt**. It's his version of a tempo run which starts at an aggressive pace and continues to get faster as it progresses. This workout does give you a good amount of time in your lactate buffering zone but it also delivers some killer mental toughness training.

Instructions:

- Just like the other tempo runs, it's beneficial to warm up for at least 2 and up to 4 miles with the first 15 minutes being at an easy pace, followed by a gradual climb in speed. Especially for this workout.

- This run is best done at level or up to 1% if that's your regular neutral incline.

- Increase the speed to your desired pace and execute for a mile.

- After a mile, increase the speed by 0.2 or more but remember the goal is to continue to increase the speed for the remaining miles.

- Once you've completed your peak mile, decrease the treadmill speed to a slow run and/or brisk walk to cool down for at least 10 minutes.

4. Downward Dog

Many running courses brag about a 'Net downhill' course which is very appealing to many runners. This provides a great opportunity to run a personal best. If you're getting ready for a course like this, it's a really good idea to do some treadmill running on a decline. Decline running also helps with your leg turnover speed which is an acquired co-ordination that you will get better at with practice. For these reasons, this workout is classified as a **speed workout**.

As stated previously, decline running causes concentric muscle contractions which happen when you hit the ground and your quads flex in an instinctive attempt to protect your joints and ligaments and slow down your momentum. As a result, this workout is **hard on your quads and knees** as well as all of the associated decline training or racing. ligaments. You will experience this for yourself in the days following your first few times attempting it. However, I firmly believe the training benefit outweighs the risk, particularly if you are training for longer distances that involve running down hills.

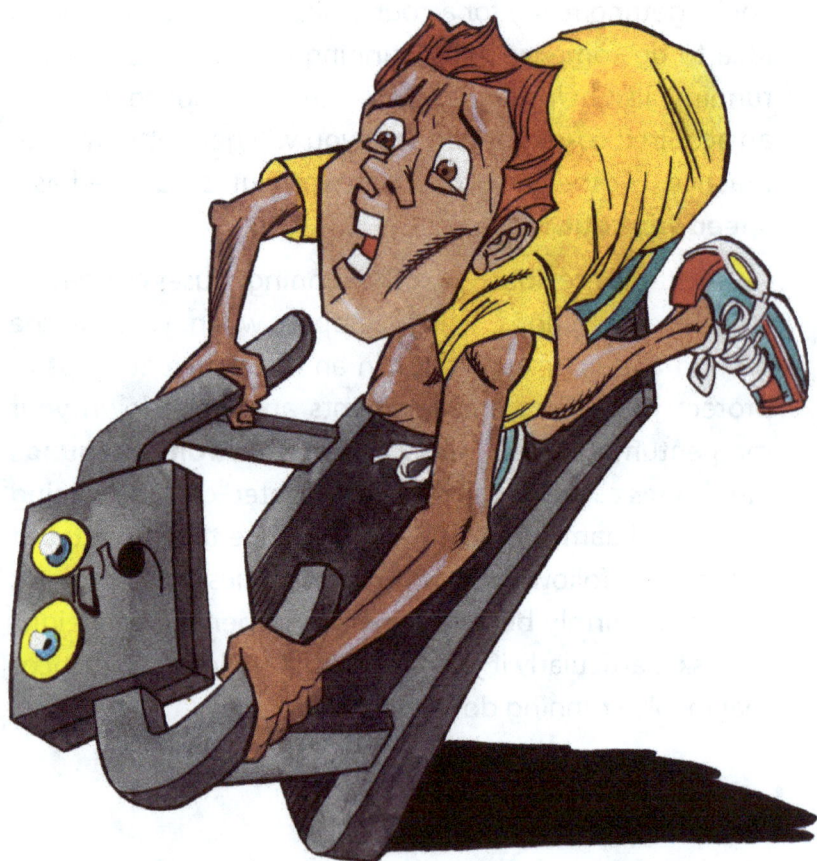

Here are a few basic tips for minimizing injury risk when executing downhill running:

1. **Be mindful of your speed. It's easy to want to pick up the pace as you run on a decline, but increased speed places more demand on your musculature.**

2. **Build your time spent on declines** *gradually* **over several weeks.**

*The following workout requires a treadmill with a decline option **OR** the use of a 2" x 6" board under the back of your treadmill to give you a -3% decline option.

Please keep in mind, that like runners, not all treadmills are alike! While I've personally had many years of flawless operation with my treadmill propped up at the back with a piece of wood, you should find out if YOUR treadmill can handle the extra stress created by the change in position. My treadmill has a hefty 4 HP motor and so you may want to consult with your treadmill manufacturer if you have any doubts about yours!

Instructions:

- After 1 to 1.5 mile warm up at your level/starting incline, drop the incline by -1%. Pace increases are optional but not recommended until you are accustomed to doing decline running.

- Hold for 5 minutes and return to level incline for 2 minutes.

- Drop the incline by -2% and hold for 5 minutes then return to level incline for 2 minutes.

- Drop the incline by -3% and hold for 5 minutes then return to level incline for another recovery of 2 minutes.

Endurance

Running marathons will require **patience**, control and inward focus - all things that training on a treadmill can provide. So many times you hear someone say, "I **hate** treadmills, they are sooooo damn boring!" Yes, they sure *can* be, and for that very reason – there is little better training to develop mental toughness for marathon day.

In any case, you'll see that doing big miles, such as those required if you perform all or most of your marathon training on a treadmill, will actually provide you with many unexpected training benefits.

Medium Long run

These are runs that range in distance between the 10 and 15 mile mark. These are a great stimulus of aerobic cellular development for runners training for endurance events such as the half or full marathon. However they are also of great benefit to build a solid foundation for runners of shorter distances. Since these running workouts are typically sandwiched in the middle of a higher volume training week, the intensity should be kept to the aerobic zone for the majority of the run.

Long run

These are the grand-daddy of all the workouts for proper endurance training preparation. Long runs typically range anywhere from 16 to 24 miles (or more) and provide a long list of training benefits that prepare you well for the demands of endurance events. In short, an endurance training program without long runs is not a training program!

To get the most benefit from your time spent doing long runs, consider breaking them down into 3 separate sections with a slightly increased pace as the run progresses. So, for example, a 15 mile medium long run would have 5 miles easy, 5 miles steady aerobic pace and 5 miles quicker than the previous 5. This keeps things interesting mentally and trains your body to expect increases in pace later in runs as you are getting tired.

Do you know your half or full marathon pace? This is an important question to answer in order to determine what an ideal pace for your long runs is. Go to www.meet-your-running-goals.com/pace-calculator.html and put in your projected half or full marathon time goal. Then select your running distance in the second box. The calculator will generate your required running pace in minutes/mile or minutes/kilometer (*see below*).

Instructions:

- All long runs should begin at any easy pace for 15 to 20 minutes followed by gradual climbs in speed.

- After warm up, increase your pace to between 1 and 1.5 minutes slower than your projected distance race pace and hold for the first third of your run (45 minutes of a 3 hour run)

- During the second portion of your long run, increase your pace to be between 1 minute and 45 seconds slower than your projected pace.

- During the last portion of your long run, increase your pace to between 45 and 30 seconds slower than your projected pace. Every few long runs, consider running the last mile or two at or close to your half or full marathon pace.

General Aerobic Workouts

These runs make up the majority of the miles within a training program. The key to these runs is staying within your aerobic zone for at least the majority of the run. Spending ample time within your aerobic zone promotes a healthy balance of fat and glycogen energy partitioning. Also, since the intensity is low to medium, recovery is minimal and your body has the opportunity to adapt quickly within this zone. To establish a good estimate of your aerobic zone, refer to the heart rate training zone page.

1. Fitness Trail

I was originally inspired by this kind of workout after running on the 'vita parcourse', or fitness trail, in Switzerland. A fitness trail is an excellent total body workout that incorporates the beauty of running with total body resistance training. It occurred to me one day, after running for 10 years on the treadmill that I had never tried to combine a total body workout with my treadmill.

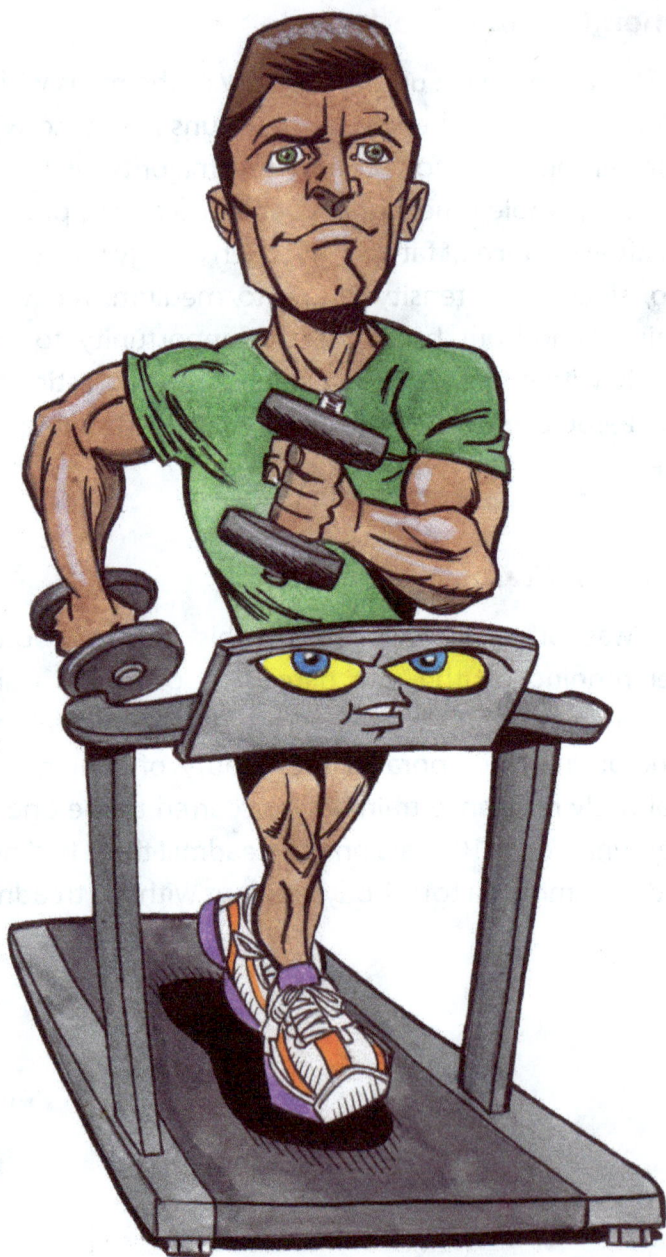

These are particularly useful training runs if you are training for a tough trail run or a combination running/obstacle course such as the increasingly popular 'Mudder' or 'Spartan' runs that will place resistance demands on your whole body. While they can be as hard as you make them, the idea is not to run aggressively during the running portion so your legs can still get a break from the continuous running of the rest of your program. For this reason, they are classified general aerobic runs.

Instructions:

- Start the treadmill at an easy pace and level incline and run for 10 to 15 minutes.

- Safely hop off the treadmill (leave it running) and do a set of **push ups** until exhaustion.

- Get back on the treadmill and run for 5 minutes.

- Safely hop off the treadmill (leave it running) and do a set of **dumbbell squats.**

- Get back on the treadmill and run for 5 minutes.

- Safely hop off the treadmill (leave it running) and do a set of **pull ups.**

- Continue to cycle through this circuit or add your favourite total body workouts to the mix.

- Cool down with at least a 5 minute brisk walk.

2. Pacing Run

Depending on the event you're training for, these workouts provide the opportunity to practice the pace that you plan to hold during the event you are training for.

For example, a half-marathon can be run at your projected marathon pace as a way to reinforce what you expect your body to do on marathon day. Pacing runs can even be done in small chunks such as the last 3 miles of a long run. The goal of the pacing run is to train to the exact pace without going too slow or fast so that it will become second nature.

Just to reiterate the goal of these runs: They are not all out race days but are goal specific pacing that occurs within an otherwise general aerobic run. So, unless they are a part of a long run, these can stay in the medium effort bucket.

Instructions:

- Start the treadmill at an easy pace and level incline and run for 10 to 15 minutes.
- Increase your pace but stay within your aerobic zone for the majority of your run.
- During the final miles of your run, increase the pace to your projected race pace.
- Cool down with 5 to 10 minutes of easy running or walking.

Running Games

The following activities are things you can incorporate into your general aerobic workout days where you otherwise have nothing special going on.

Mind over Matter – observe your heart rate as you run without reducing your pace. Work at taking deeper, slower breaths and running with a very relaxed posture while maintaining good running from. Focus on your heart rate coming down. I find that thinking of a peaceful place (my happy place) helps me to relax. Observe your heart rate slowly fall. See how low you can get it. You will be surprised!

Speedplay (fartlek)/Strides – these are essentially little bursts of speed thrown into your regular aerobic pace runs where you focus on good running form. The idea is for them to be rather impulsive and have very little structure. After a good warm up period, once you've settled into your run, increase the belt pace and hold for no more than 30 seconds. You can do the same for incline by playing with your up and downs. Just remember to keep your bursts short because it's not supposed to be a true interval run.

Gonzalez – This one will sound weird, I know, but I like doing it and some of you might too. You must be **very** careful with this one as it can be dangerous if you don't execute it properly. This is a pure leg turn over drill where you support most of your weight on the side bars (assuming you have them). After a good warm up period, hop on your side rails and crank the treadmill to max speed.

Yes, max speed. Holding up most of your weight on the side bars, let your feet lightly touch the belt as it screams by. Try and keep up with the pace, as soon as you become tired (either triceps or legs) hop back onto the side rails for a quick recovery.

Recovery Workouts

These ideally low intensity and low distance runs are a method of active recovery following a higher intensity workout or race. Rather than sit around and do nothing, recovery runs help to promote blood flow to areas with inflammation. Great care must be taken to properly warm up and keep the pace down throughout the entire run. Following up with gentle stretching routine can be of great benefit to loosen things up as well. I don't have any interesting runs to prescribe for recovery days, but rather just a small soapbox lecture to say:

- Keep the pace and incline down.
- Don't be afraid to walk.
- Don't think twice about taking a day off if you are sore.
- If you perform a cross training activity that involves your legs, keep the intensity low.

·D·

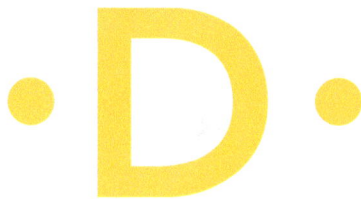

GET POSITIVE RESULTS

So far we've looked at the importance of setting great goals that are meaningful, challenging yet realistic for you. We've looked at a variety of inexpensive ways that you can enhance your workout environment to create positive running experiences. We also explored many stimulating tools that are available to help making running on the treadmill a fun and effective training tool.

The fourth and equally crucial pillar that contributes to your long term motivation is staying healthy and getting results. Any progress from your starting point is very encouraging to help you stay focussed and continue working toward your goals.

We all get discouraged if we think that we aren't getting results from our hard work and it makes perfect sense. We should expect to get returns from the worthy pursuit of our goals. This is why it's both important to ensure that your goals are measurable in the first place as well as take the time to measure your progress to make sure you are on the right track.

TAP INTO DAILY ENERGY

"Do the thing and you shall get the energy to do the thing".

B. Proctor

Many of you may get this far and think, *Well, okay, I have great and ambitious goals, my treadmill is in a stimulating environment but my problem is I'm just so busy and tired all the time. I have a hard time getting my butt on the treadmill after a long day at work.*

Getting different results often involves doing things in a different way. To maximize your chances of having the energy to even start your workout, review, and give serious and honest consideration to, the following things that can have a profound effect on your energy levels:

- Eating the Right Calories
- Sleep
- Hydration

DEREK LALONDE

SMART EATING

Eating right is critical to your long term success and makes a big difference on your energy levels day to day. I'll be the first to admit that I've fallen off the wagon, as many times if not more than anyone in this category. However, I do pay the price, particularly if I'm in heavy training for an upcoming run.

The quality, frequency and amount of calories you take in every time you eat a meal will have a direct impact on your blood sugar and therefore your energy levels. Likewise, an over stimulated nervous system due to excessive caffeine intake will have also have a big impact on your energy levels.

I believe that I would be extremely remiss if I didn't take the time to put a BIG magnifying glass to the heart of the matter when it comes to how important what you eat is to your success as far as getting results from your training. Let's face it many, if not most, people got into running in the first place because a change was needed in lifestyle and/or in body composition.

I've always been a firm believer, that the best way to lose weight is by walking and running your way toward a clear goal rather than by focusing on losing weight. It's also important to understand that your weight, and more importantly body composition, is closely related to your running performance.

What this means in a nutshell is that a lean, mean, great looking body that has been carved out by training and proper nutrition will not only look and feel great to you, it will help you to meet your running goals.

So let's look at a few key **FACTS** about training, diet and the nutrition.

Consuming the right food, at the right time will:

1. **Help you to recover from training in order to get stronger and faster by providing glycogen replacement and aiding in muscle repair.**

2. **Help you to maintain stable blood sugar levels throughout the day for consistent workout energy.**

3. **Help you to get positive results both in body composition changes and running performance.**

Anyone who thinks that what you eat is either less than half or some smaller percent of the picture is dead WRONG! In fact, instead of thinking about diet and exercise as an *equal partnership*, it's more accurate to think of your nutrition intake as the **foundation** that you build exercise upon.

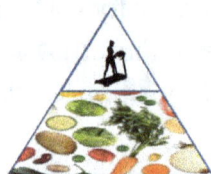

Without a strong foundation of diet, you're at high risk for going nowhere fast on your treadmill. Don't get me wrong, you will still experience a degree of results and change, but nothing near what your body and running performance can be!

In addition to the above listed reasons as to why it's so important to make sure that you get your nutrition right, runners can be at an even higher risk than sedentary people to overeat and/or consume the wrong calories. This results due to a phenomenon known as 'reward eating'. We have all done it – and here's how it works.

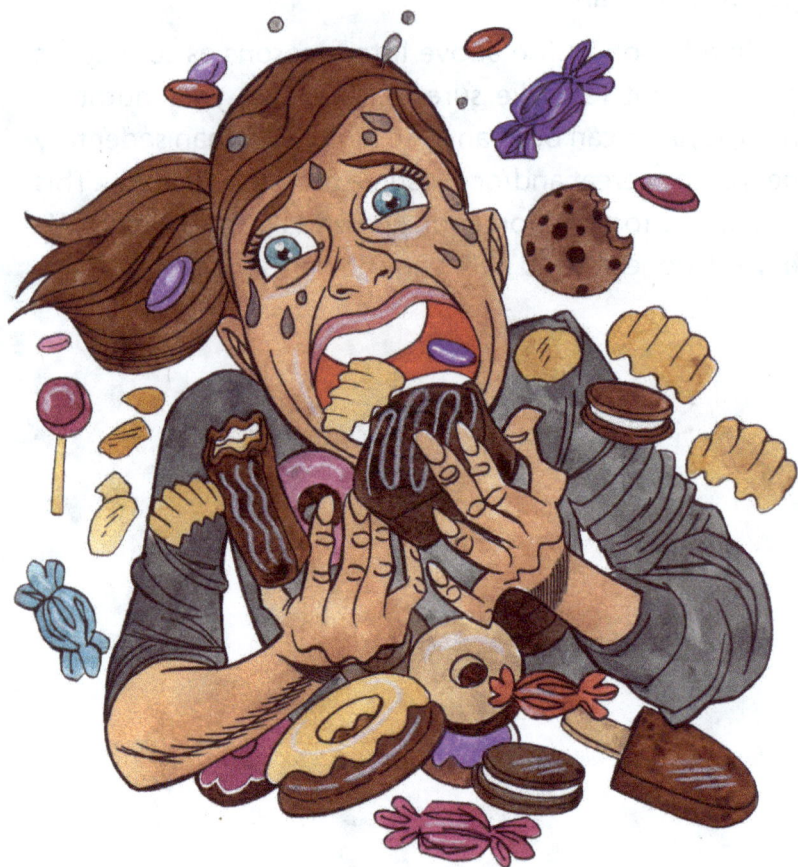

You are a good Doobie and you get your run in for the day. You get off the treadmill famished and find yourself in the kitchen quickly stuffing whatever is easy and accessible into your mouth during your post-run stretch routine. There happens to be an open bag of chips in the pantry. "Oh great, well, I need salt so these won't hurt. Some dark chocolate? Yes, I'll eat that too, I heard that's chalk full of antioxidants and other good stuff.

It's not that these indulgences are such a bad thing if consumed in moderation and perhaps at other times, but they are not the nutrient rich calories your body craves and needs after a workout. So your hunger signal stays on urging you to consume more and more.

Some people will use the completion of the weekly long run as an excuse to binge drink the rest of the weekend (ahem).

Over the course of a 12 to 18 week training program, these kinds of habits can really take their toll, including a noticeable lack of results. And we have an uncanny way of justifying these actions while outwardly we are perplexed that we actually gained weight after working so hard for so long! The bottom line is your workout isn't done until you're off the treadmill and you've consumed a nutritious post-workout shake.

Next to the treadmill, my favourite machine in the house is my *juicer*. If you're not already into juicing, give this some serious consideration. Juicers range in price starting from around $100 and can go up to about $400. In my humble opinion, the two main attributes to look for when considering which model to buy in order of importance (not unlike treadmills) is the **power** of the unit followed by the ease of cleaning after use.

This is my favourite post hard workout juice:

- 1 bunch of kale
- 2 carrots
- 1 beet
- 1 orange
- 1 apple
- 1 lemon

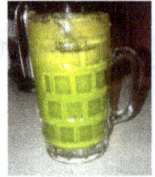

This produces a light green and surprisingly great tasting beverage that's nutritionally loaded including a huge healthy dose of vitamin C to manage post-exercise free radical damage.

Of course, the beauty of juicing is you can experiment with all kinds of produce to get different flavours (and colours). The best part is your body is immediately receiving bioavailable nutrients in the right way at the right time.

There are a few reasons this is so good for you:

- Quality weight loss takes time and occurs as a result of a combination of diet and exercise. Getting rid of the post-workout binge is a key component of long-term success.

- Eating properly, in addition to consistent balanced

training, will get you the best results. And getting great results is how you stay motivated to keep working toward future goals.

Hydration

Enough cannot be said about keeping yourself hydrated with clean water! This is one of the single most important things you can do to help your performance, beat running fatigue and boost your overall energy level. Your body relies on water for so many of its vital functions and it's the key to feeling good. Do your best to get into the habit of having water bottles easily accessible at home, in the car, at the office. Half the battle is having water around to reach for anytime, anywhere. The next time you're feeling beat by running fatigue and low on energy, reconsider that cup of coffee and go for a great big glass of water!

Workout Time

We are all individuals with our own unique set of genetics in addition to our life routine. If you experiment with running at different times of the day, you will find that there are certain periods where you will naturally have more energy and better runs than others. For example, in addition to being an early riser some people are very sensitive to the impact that daylight has on their body. In this case, running in the evening might be quite an arduous task compared to figuring out how to schedule it earlier in the day.

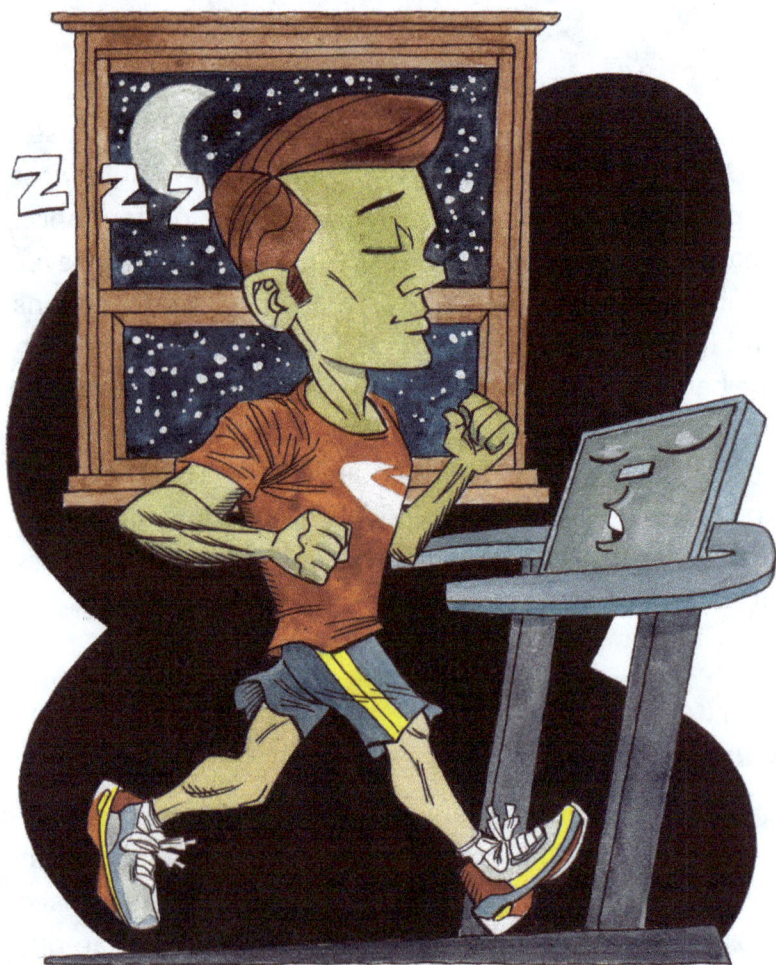

Others have fantastic runs later in the day. I personally find that later in the morning to lunch time to be my sweet spot. Experiment as much as possible with working out at different times of the day and you'll likely find the time that works best with your biology. While your body is quite adaptive, you might do well to at least perform your high intensity workouts, such as intervals and tempo runs, during your more suitable 'finest hours'. This is where having a treadmill in your house is a real bonus.

One other thing to remember though, is the point of training is to prepare you for a specific performance goal. If your half marathon will take place at 8:00 AM on a Sunday morning (which most do), you should mirror this workout time at least in the weeks leading up to your run.

Sleep

Many runners underestimate the increased need for sleep relative to their training volume. Being in a bedtime and morning routine that allows for a fixed amount of sleep (i.e. 7 hours) it's easy to fall into gradual sleep deprivation mode. Look at changing small things like watching TV or your laptop in bed or whatever it takes to squeeze in extra sleep time. You'll have more energy for your daily runs, be more likely to stay off the injury list and enjoy better performance all around.

Remember though, that recovery isn't just about what you eat and how easy you take the day after a hard workout. Quality recovery takes place when you **SLEEP!**

If you train consistently you need to be consistently careful about getting adequate sleep, or you may experience one, or all, of these issues:

- Performance declines
- Depressed immune system
- Higher risk of injury
- Cranky disposition
- Loss of motivation

According to Dr. John Conforti, Internist, Pulmonolgoist and Sleep Medicine Specialist, athletes need to better understand and appreciate what's happening to their body when they sleep. *"**Many hormones are actually released during sleep and at different stages of sleep. Some are reparative; some are for new cell growth. Growth hormones such as cortisol, leptin and greylin actually effect appetite and glucose control. Also, not to mention the fact that it's very difficult to run well when you're physically exhausted.**"*

As we all know, the challenges with getting enough sleep while working hard to meet your goals in the middle of a busy work and family life are many. Add to this the very bizarre and unwavering tendency of our society to associate sleeping in with guilt. For anyone who tries to guilt you for getting 'too much' sleep, invite them to set goals and train along with you. If you are someone who feels guilty for getting a long restful night of sleep by going to bed early, it's time to get over it! Your body will thank you in a variety of ways including an improved running performance.

Here are a few basic tips to help you get a better night's sleep:

1. **Keep evening workouts low key – s**everal studies suggest that evening workouts don't necessarily have a negative impact on your ability to fall asleep and have a restful sleep. However, try to avoid the really taxing workouts such as intervals or threshold runs as these are very stimulating to your nervous system.

2. **Take control of your devices –** laptops and handhelds have completely invaded every aspect of our lives including the bedroom. It's just too easy to watch a movie or surf in bed. If that's something you love to do, get to bed earlier to make up for the activity, and be strict about the time to close it up.

3. **Limit your caffeine and alcohol intake after supper -** Both substances can hinder a restful sleep.

4. **Nap at the right time -** short naps (10 to 20 minutes) are an awesome way to recharge during the day or late afternoon but evening naps can be disastrous. Try to get to bed early rather than nap late.

5. **Get serious about sleep, but don't stress about loss of sleep!** - We all experience it from time to time. Just like your training and diet, sleep deprivation is more of a chronic problem rather than an issue of one or two nights. So, it's what you can do 85% of the time that matters. Also keep in mind that 37.5% of all statistics are made up :)

DAILY MOTIVATION TIP*

Yet another strategy to help you get your run in on one of those crazy days, which we all have now and again, is to simply agree with yourself to commit to start!

An unexpected recovery day is definitely not the end of the world, nor will it matter in the big picture in your program. It might even help. But to ensure it's your body telling you to take a break and not your brain, commit to a 20 minute warm up period. That's it and that's all. If after 20 minutes, you still feel like the tank is empty, can it for the day.

Sometimes we focus too much on the end results rather than what is immediately in front of us.

Half the battle of getting your run in is making the time to do it, including changing into your running clothes and just beginning. I'm willing to bet at least half of the time, or more, that you employ this strategy you'll end up getting your run done.

Sticking to a program successfully requires you to get emotionally attached to your goal and helps you to be driven. This drive is very healthy and necessary to your success, but at the same time it becomes difficult to take that unplanned day off. If you commit to the warm up, which will require you to change, put the time aside and get your butt on the treadmill. At least you can say you really made an honest effort to get it done.

DEREK LALONDE

THE ART OF WARMING UP

Probably the most humbling running lesson I've ever learned, and many runners make this mistake, is starting your runs too fast. True, this mistake will have devastating effects on race day, but many a training run are ruined this way too. Without exception, regardless of your experience level, warming up should be treated in a sacred fashion.

Many top runners walk briskly or run at least 2 minutes per mile slower than their anticipated running pace for the day during the warm up period. Before you even get going, you can entertain some ballistic stretching to get things warmed up and pliable. Slow starts also give your body time to establish energy partitioning where it decides what energy will be coming from where. Easier early paces help your body to tap into your body fat stores rather than use your muscle glycogen for energy. Burning a good balance of the two greatly contributes to a solid amount of long term energy while you run.

Easing into your runs provides the opportunity for your cardiovascular and muscular system to getting warmed up which will help to avoid injury. If you're an experienced runner, you will know the value of a good warm up before a workout of any intensity. This strategy not only helps to prevent an acute injury, it also greatly increases your chances of having a great workout. This is because as mentioned above, a gradual warm up will maximize your chances of burning a well balanced mix of carbs and fat which should translate into lasting longer and feeling better for the duration of your run.

You either already know from experience, or have heard from other runners, that you'll rarely have a great training run when you haven't properly warmed up. Whether you are planning to run a short and high intensity workout or intend to be out for a 3 hour run, start SLOW and give your body ample time to warm up. Ample time typically means at least 15 to 20 minutes of anywhere from a very brisk walk to a light jog.

Despite best efforts, we all experience the odd day where we feel like we're running low on energy reserves, but don't let it get you down. Perhaps you're not being whiny, and your body would much rather do with a brisk walk! Listen to your body and try to enjoy your session for whatever it brings and be proud of yourself for getting off your butt. Hydrate, consume some quality calories, get a good night's sleep and resume with a fresh start the next day.

THE RUNNER'S HIGH

If your workouts are more often enjoyable experiences, you are much more likely to look forward to repeating them.

The term 'runner's high' is used to describe the sensation that is experienced due to the endorphin release brought on by running. I've also heard of it referred to as a runner's orgasm. Your pituitary gland releases endorphins in response to stress, or any kind of pain, experienced by the body. While this endorphin release is not exclusively experienced by runners, the runner's high is brought on as a result of the stress caused by running for a period of time. Keep in mind that stress, particularly stress induced by exercise such as running, is both healthy to impose on your body and essential for adaptation, growth and progress.

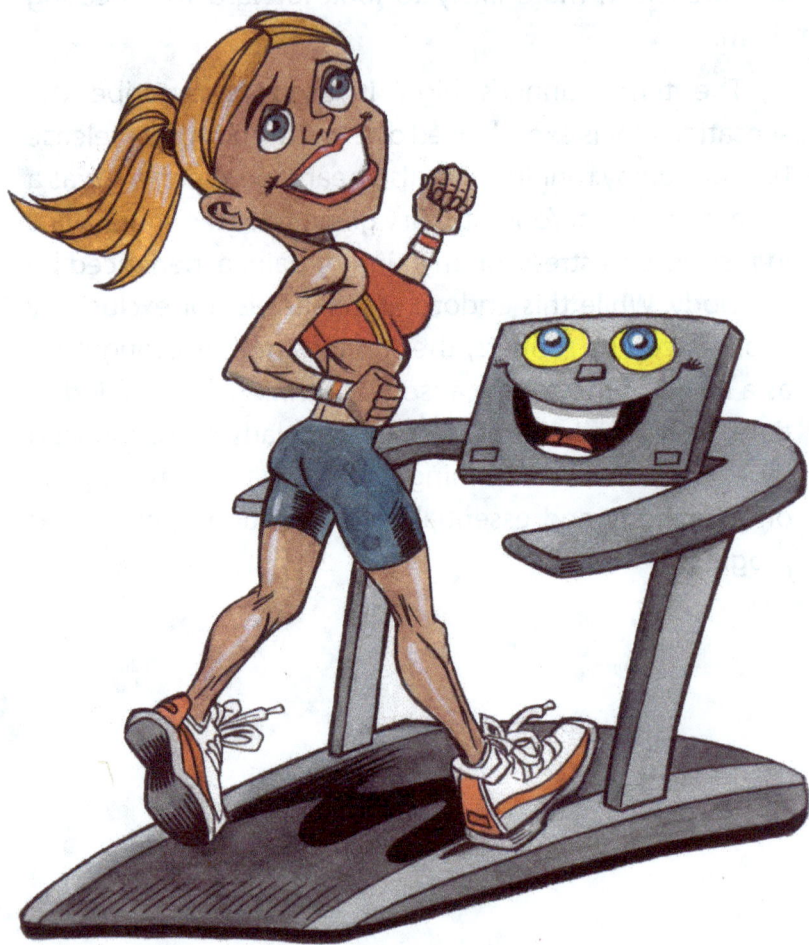

There are a few interesting facts about a runner's high that you might not have known. Some runners experience the high much earlier, as early as 10 minutes, while others may not experience the high until several hours into a run. This might be the reason why many beginner runners don't report experiencing a runner's high, they simply aren't running long enough!

Without much hard scientific evidence, I can only draw from the vast number of runners who report a runner's high. But among those runners, the time and sensation differs depending on the distances. Specifically, distance runners who regularly run 16 to 22 miles seem to experience runner's high much later in their runs than those who typically run much less. It's personally quite common for me to feel a sudden sense of well-being during my second or even third hour of a long run. Some describe this as a 'second wind'.

This likely has much to do with the adaptation that has taken place in the body of the distance runner over time. Since they are more used to running for longer than 1 hour, the perceived stress of running on the body might be much less than that of a shorter distance runner. That said, higher intensity runs of any kind such as track workouts or hill repeats also will trigger the endorphin release.

Experiencing a runner's high is a wonderful and healthful feeling and it only makes sense that ideally everyone would want to experience this during every run. This, however, doesn't seem to be the case. I've heard of countless runners complaining that they 'may' have experienced runner's high but they certainly don't experience it very often, if at all.

Through diligent training logs kept over the years including such comments as 'invigorating, felt great today, finished strong', along with some basic principles of exercise physiology, I've been able to identify a pattern of key actions that increase your chances of experiencing runner's high more frequently.

*Tips to Experience Runner's High More Frequently

The first strategy is to pay very close attention to your **warm up!** The second strategy is to ensure that you are **not running on empty**. Make sure that you are fuelled before your run and also have enough water and glycogen sources with you for the duration of the run. If your body is in a depleted state, you will feel crappy and no amount of endorphins will do much for you.

Wherever possible, **remove any sources of discomfort**. This includes being overdressed or underdressed for the conditions you will be running in or worse, under-lubed! Much like being under-'caloried', being uncomfortable during your run due to heat, cold or friction will greatly diminish your ability to enjoy your endorphin release.

Another key strategy to get that runner's high is to pursue **high intensity interval training**. While a runner's high is not reliant on high intensity, fast-paced running, doing the same pace every day will eventually do little to stimulate or 'stress' your body. This is due to adaptation and will therefore limit your chances for a nice runner's high. Little comes close to the feeling you will experience after a well-executed fartlek session, a good hard bout of intervals or hill repeats !

DEREK LALONDE

SMART TRAINING

It's not enough to follow a well-balanced program, if you're not mindful of how much effort you are putting into your workouts.

Heart rate training is an excellent way to get the most out of every workout for athletes of ALL levels. Heart rate running training might very well be the smartest and most effective thing you can do for your running progress. Training by heart rate is not only an objective way of controlling your running intensities; it's also a very effective way of monitoring how well your body is responding to your training. Listening to your heart rather than going by feel removes your personal judgement from the mix and tells a true story.

Most treadmills come equipped with the ability to display heart rate during your workout. There are a variety of ways they can do this such as via the metal grip on the side handle bars. It's hard though not to interrupt a good running groove to place and keep your hands on the side bars to get your heart rate so the much more convenient option is to wear a chest strap. If your treadmill did not come with a chest strap, a heart rate monitor that can transmit to your phone or sometimes plug into your machine directly are options to consider.

DEREK LALONDE

HEART RATE TRAINING ZONES

Find your heart rate training zone for each type of workout by using either scientific or more crude, but effective, methods. There is a heart rate training zone that is dedicated to every kind of running workout. We've all heard the credo, **'Train smarter not harder.'** But what does that really mean?

Paying attention to your exercise heart rate while training, ensures that in your training program, your efforts are properly placed. You want to make sure that you are running easy/moderate pace on the days that you should be so that you have more to give to the designated **HARD** days in your program. Basically, finding out what your heart rate training zones are, and then paying attention to what is going on during your workouts, optimizes your adaptation and minimizes your risk for injury. This is what training smarter is all about!

For me, a heart rate monitor often keeps me from going too hard on 'recovery' days. Those days where you feel great but your heart says, "I'm tired!" A very effective way to avoid over training is to regularly **check your resting heart rate.**

A simple and effective method to check your resting heart rate is during the exact moment you open your eyes in the morning before you get out of bed. Slowly, place your first and second finger on your neck and count the number of heart beats in a minute. Use your bedroom clock for measurement. You can also use a heart rate monitor if you remember to leave it on your nightstand. If you get into the habit of checking your resting heart rate over the weeks and months of training, you'll gain a good sense of how your body is responding and recovering to your program stimulus. You'll also likely notice a dropping resting heart rate over time as your heart becomes stronger and more efficient at pumping blood as indicated by a lower resting heart rate.

What are the Heart Rate Training Zones?

While some people have a different numbering system for the training zones, I've provided an explanation below for each one in this context. Basically, in terms of pace, the various training zones can be described as:

- **Zone 0**: Easy/Recovery
- **Zone 1**: Moderate General Aerobic – most miles
- **Zone 2**: Steady pace (marathon race pace)
- **Zone 3**: Anaerobic threshold/lactate buffering – point at which lactate in muscles continues to rise
- **Zone 4**: VO2 max
- **Zone 5**: Red zone

Roughly translated, with slight variations from individual to individual, here is another way of putting it:

- **Zone 0** - 55% - 65% of Maximum Heart Rate (MHR)
- **Zone 1** - 66% - 75% of MHR

- **Zone 2** - 76% - 80% of MHR
- **Zone 3** - 81% - 87 % of MHR
- **Zone 4** - 88% - 94% of MHR
- **Zone 5** - >95% of MHR

Notice that these zones are all based on a simple percentage calculation of your maximum heart rate!

Your true maximum heart rate, despite popular belief, is actually quite unique to you. We've all seen suggested training zones based on age graded averages at your local gym on posters and on treadmills. However these are based on maximum heart rates calculated by ***population norms***.

Therefore, if you don't currently know yours, keep reading about the various methods you can explore to establish your true maximum heart rate.

How to Find Your Heart Rate Zones

As you'll see on the heart rate zone page, there are a few ways, some easier and less expensive and hence less accurate than others.

Once you've established your maximum heart rate, you can then find your heart rate training zones by referring to my target heart rate chart. If you end up getting the step test, you'll have all of your ideal zones provided to you as part of your test!

Your Maximum Heart Rate

Your maximum heart rate is genetically determined and while it does typically decline with age in sedentary people, active athletes such as runners usually enjoy much less of a decline if any at all.

Your MHR, simply put, is the maximum rate at which your heart is currently capable of beating. This rate is most commonly expressed in terms of beats per minute (bpm). While your MHR is not an indicator of your fitness or fitness potential, it is really good to know what it is in order to establish proper heart rate training zones. Most training zones are based on a % calculation of your MHR. For example, your ideal aerobic zone for running generally falls between 55% and 65% of your MHR.

As a runner, if you plan to monitor your heart rate during training, which of course is a brilliant idea, finding out your maximum heart rate is absolutely necessary. The big reason for this is your MHR is a unique figure to you as an individual. Your max can vary or 5 to 15 beats lower or higher than average so keep that in mind.

The problem this presents is when you train by heart rate and you've established heart rate training zones based on a guess, you risk either running too slow or too fast for the goal of any given workout. When you're running too slow, your heart rate will not be high enough to benefit from a training effect. When you're running too fast, you will also miss out the opportunities for growth intended by your prescribed workout and put yourself at risk of overtraining and injury.

How to Find Your Maximum Heart Rate

There are a few ways that you can go about finding your MHR - from most crude to most accurate.

Test 1 – Standard age-graded maximum heart rate calculations available such as:

1. **220 – your age**
2. **205.8 – (0.685 × age)**

These and other similar calculations can be quite inaccurate since there is great variation from individual to individual. For the first formula, it's been found that there is a standard deviation of 11 beats per minute or more. For example, mine is **9** beats lower than this calculation. A training partner of mine is 12 beats higher than what is considered 'normal' for her age.

The second calculation is more widely accepted in the exercise physiology community as it has shown to have an average deviation of around 6 bpm. While this doesn't sound like a big deal, both errors can mean the difference between exercising properly in your 'zone 3' or wasting your time tearing yourself down. We are all unique in our specific:

- Physiology
- History
- Running Goals
- Maximum Heart Rate

So while this method of estimating your max HR takes very little time, effort and cost it's clearly not your best route.

Test 2 – Maximum Effort 'stress' Test (crude, but better than above)

A somewhat structured stress test such as a warm up followed by hill/incline sprints. There are many ways to do this test but basically you are pushed to your perceived exercise limit while wearing a heart rate monitor. **This type of test should always be administered by a trained fitness professional to ensure the safety of the runner.** You would be surprised how much further you can push when someone is yelling at you!

This test can yield pretty accurate results within a few beats per minute and will very quickly give you an idea as to whether your maximum heart rate is below, on par or much greater than the average for your age.

Test 3 – Treadmill Step Test

This test is actually designed to determine all of your training zones based on your body's blood lactate buffering capabilities. Obtaining your maximum heart rate is only one piece of the data that is collected. A runner is put through a series of paces that gradually increase. Blood samples are taken at the end of each 'stage' before the pace is increased. By measuring your blood lactate levels, the tester is able to determine various biomarkers that reflect metabolic responses in your body. These, in turn, help to establish proper training zones for your ideal development and progress.

This test can be quite expensive (between $120 and $175) and should always be administered by an able exercise technician in a laboratory setting **but** it's by far the most accurate way to find your true maximum heart rate and also your heart rate training zones.

If you're really serious about improving as a runner and think that you will get tested often or as a group, you might consider your own hand held blood lactate analyzer. I own the 'lactate pro' and am very happy with it.

DEREK LALONDE

WHAT TO MEASURE AND HOW

There are a few points worth highlighting when it comes to measuring results, particularly for runners. It's important to recognize these points so that you don't fall into the trap of getting discouraged and losing motivation on the journey toward your goals.

First, recognize that not all results will be easily measurable or observable along the way. Know that your body will grow stronger and fitter in response to the right training stimulus placed upon it. This is called the law of adaptation and in order for it to work, it requires stress followed by ample recovery time. However, adaptation occurs in stages where there are gains (or losses) followed by periods of stabilization and even resistance. The way exercise physiologists have described this phenomenon has always made me think of a slinky or spiral. You'll have periods of growth and progress followed by periods of static recovery as your body gets ready for stronger training stimuli.

While progress can be slow and steady there can even be some downward turns before the next bit of progress. It's important to recognize that your body is very dynamic when it comes to its response to training and that positive change takes consistent training, patience and time. So the lesson is, don't measure your progress too often or you may risk becoming demotivated by an apparent lack of results.

Second, measure the right variables at the right time. While 'weight' loss is pretty observable and can change fairly consistently over the course of weeks, running performance improvements and healthy body composition changes actually take longer. This is because scales don't reveal the total picture of what's going on inside the body. Dehydration or water retention can account for 3 to 5 pounds up or down depending on the circumstances. Try not to get hung up on weighing yourself unless you're attempting to monitor your fluid loss after a long run. Rather than measuring your progress with a scale, consider other healthier metrics like how your clothes fit.

Remember though, that your actual fitness progress is the most relevant metric for your objective which is to meet your running goals. I'm a big fan of training by heart rate, and one of the reasons for this is your fitness progress is easily measurable and observable over the weeks and months as your training progresses.

At the beginning of your program, you may be running 6 miles per hour on the treadmill with a heart rate of 143, and 5 weeks later the same pace with a heart rate of 135. As you become fitter and more efficient at running, your heart does not have to work as hard to create the same output as it did 5 weeks earlier. This is a clear indication of successful adaptation to training stimulus.

Changes in your fitness level as reflected by metrics such as your resting and exercise heart rate are the best measurements to monitor over the weeks and months as these are crystal clear.

Third if you are sure that you are off track, be open and willing to adjust your course or change your strategy. This last point requires you to be **brutally** honest with yourself. Often you won't know how well your training went until you run the event at the end of your program. However, **every** run provides you with an opportunity for learning something about yourself.

DEREK LALONDE

WHAT TO LOOK FOR IN A TREADMILL

If you are currently, or may soon be, in the market for a new or replacement treadmill, this chapter is for you. If, on the other hand, you already own a treadmill or work out in a gym, you could probably care less and may want to *skip to the next chapter.*

A friend of mine who owned a local fitness equipment retailer for many years once shared a little known trade secret with me when it came to treadmills. He told me that most residential treadmill models are not actually designed to take the pounding of running. If they were actually used as much as people intended when they bought them, the companies would quickly go out of business with warranty work as the machines would start to show signs of wear fairly early in their lifespan. When I first heard this news, I was shocked. How could this actually be true? With so many promises of versatility, power and assuring warranty options, surely these machines can live up to their longevity claims!

Apparently not. My friend went on to explain that, much like the sales of gym memberships, many people make these purchases with the best of intentions and start out by using their treadmills quite regularly. Eventually, and often within a fairly short period of time, the machines become clothes racks somewhere in a desolate spot in the basement. This, of course, does not describe you, which is why you have this book and also why you need to ensure that you get a treadmill that is actually designed to handle the stresses of running!

With this in mind, if you are in the market for a treadmill, and you actually intend to use that treadmill as the powerful running training tool that it can be, you must be aware of what to look for.

Here are some of the key points to consider when you're in the market for a treadmill, starting with the most important:

1. The Strong Silent Type (Horse Power!)

A treadmill should be seen as a long term investment that can bring you countless hours of worry-free effective training. You might currently be a newer runner training a few times a week in which case a certain model of treadmill may meet your needs. But it's also important when selecting the right treadmill that you look down the road to what your **future** running and training needs may be. As crazy as it may seem at the present, you should think of your treadmill as a training tool that can take the beating of marathon or even ultra-marathon training. This might mean daily use including runs lasting several hours at a time. You will also need to think about your machine being able to handle the various types of workouts that any good training program will require of you including short, long, slow, fast, flat or hilly runs and any combination of these.

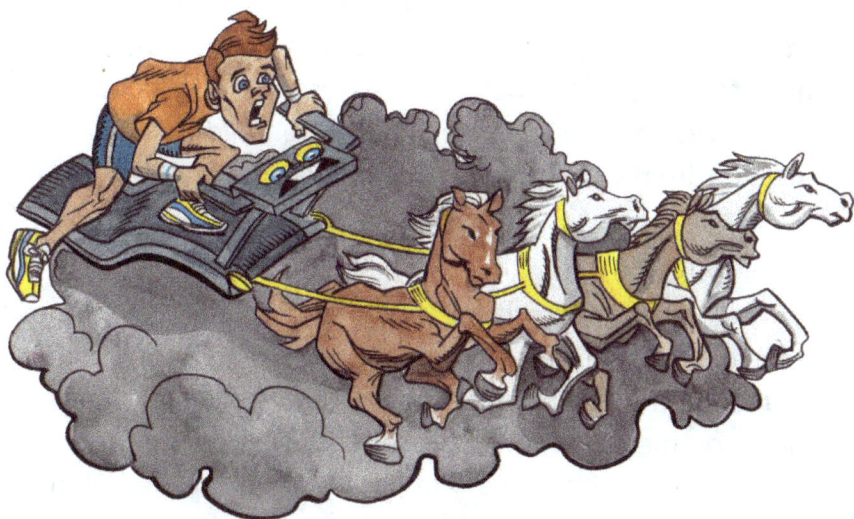

All this to say when picking a treadmill the most important component that will determine whether or not it can handle all the stresses of a dynamic training program is the size of the motor under the hood and its ability to provide **continuous horse power (CHP) also referred to as continuous duty power (CDP)** versus intermittent horsepower delivery power without overheating.

This basically describes how much uninterrupted power a treadmill can deliver during use. When the treadmill speed is increased, this places a demand on the motor to increase the belt speed in response. The demand for increased belt speed is higher if the treadmill is at an incline with the weight of a runner.

A high CHP delivers the necessary power to accommodate the increases with little to no hesitation experienced by the runner. Higher CHP motors have the ability to handle heavier runners under similar stressful situations without bogging down. Higher CHP machines are also able to respond to user changes much quicker. This feature becomes really important when you're doing intervals and need to get from 5 to 9 miles per hour as quickly as possible to simulate outdoor track conditions.

The better residential treadmills that will easily handle the demands of hard-core treadmill runners have at least a **3** CHP motor. Even if you plan to mostly walk on the treadmill, using steep inclines at a brisk walking pace places decent demands on the motor so don't opt for anything less than a 2.5 Continuous Duty motor.

The motor of a treadmill is really in a class of its own in importance. There is no point in having any other great components without a great motor for support.

The bottom line is CONTINUOUS HORSE POWER IS KING! You will **never** regret having more horsepower than you need.

2. Roller Bearings

Bearings are the heart of the long cylindrical devices that look like giant rolling pins at the front and back of your treadmill. High quality bearings are typically 2" or more in diameter and have excellent seals that keep out dirt and grit while holding in grease for smooth movement. The size of the bearings and their seals are super important features as they contribute to proper belt tracking, tension and minimum friction. Usually high horse power machines will accompany heavier duty rollers and bearings, but it's worth inquiring to be sure.

3. Ease of Use

Many treadmills have built-in programs designed to challenge you with various aspects of targeted fitness which can be fun and convenient, however you'll really appreciate the option to just hop on a treadmill and get going with full and easy control over the speed and incline. So, the first thing to look for is a very obvious **quick start** button.

A second important component of the start and stop buttons, as well as the speed and incline buttons, is their size and sensitivity. You want buttons that are big and easy enough to hit on the fly but definitely not too sensitive to hit by accident.

4. Incline & Top Speed

Well-designed treadmills can be used by athletes of any level. Even if you are choosing a treadmill to predominantly walk on, anticipate the possibility of running in the future. Likewise, runners should dream big when it comes to top speed. Something like 10 mph may sound like more than you'll ever need but you would really be disappointed if you discover that you can't do more if you wanted to without buying a better machine!

At risk of sounding cliché, your current situation does not necessarily dictate your future results. In other words, expect great progress from yourself and get more incline and top speed than you think you need today. Incline and top speed go hand in hand with bigger motors so if you get sufficient horse power, these top end features should be there.

5. The Long Pause

This is the amount of time your treadmill will stay in a holding pattern if you happen to pause in the middle of your workout. Think about having to hit the bathroom in the middle of your run, and not wanting to lose your stats (time, distance and calories).

This feature may seem silly, and possibly not something you can necessarily add as a feature, but I would wager you would really learn to appreciate it. When working out on gym treadmills, I would have to sprint to get to the bathroom and back in time in order to keep my place because this hold time was so short. My current treadmill which is the Landice L7 Residential unit has what appears to be an indefinite pause feature which I have really grown to appreciate over time.

These are the most important features to consider when you are comparing treadmill models to buy.

Other things that matter...but less

Like the frame and drive train of a car, quality is important to look for, but not something you'll necessarily notice or that you will wish you had while using your machine. But there are features you'll find contribute to your daily enjoyment of the treadmill.

Also, it's worth giving consideration to what each of these features cost versus what you are actually getting (a cost/benefit analysis) to get the right machine at a price that suits your budget.

1. Deck length

Deck Length is more about preference than necessity as most runners tend not to drift too much from the front console during running. As long as you have enough room to freely swing your arms without coming into contact with the console you will adapt to pretty much any length of deck. If you are an over-strider or particularly tall and find that you need the extra length to stretch out during your run it may mean a bit more to you. However, you would gain much more benefit from improving your running form to minimize over-striding rather than accommodate it!

2. Heart Rate Monitor

A heart rate monitor feature is actually a fantastic option to have. However, it is not absolutely essential for this feature to be built into your treadmill. As a runner, if you don't already have a heart rate monitor/watch, you should seriously look at obtaining one whether you run on a treadmill or not. In which case, you won't need to have one built into your treadmill. Just like other extra options on a treadmill, take the time to look at what the extra cost is for the option. A decent heart rate monitor with a watch and chest strap can be acquired for under $100 which you can use on and off of the treadmill. I personally have had many good years with Polar HR monitors.

3. Belt Thickness

The thickness of the tread belt is not so much something you'll notice while running but higher quality belts are thicker and therefore last much longer than thinner ones. Belt ply thickness is one way that cheaper treadmills differ from more expensive ones. Cheaper belts will be 1 or 2 ply where better models sport up to 4 ply belt thickness.

4. Frame/Treadmill Weight

This really comes down to what kind of space you have available in your home or apartment. You want a stable, heavy enough frame so that you're not shaking and wobbling all over the place. If you need a machine that you plan on folding/rolling into place every time you use it, you will need to look at some lighter portable options. Just know that this will mean a little less stability when in use. The big heavy models are a pain to move but worth the weight once they are in place.

5. Emergency Stop

I realize this won't be a popular thing to say, but as a hard-core treadmill user, emergency stop buttons have been the cause of more frustrations on treadmills than anything else I've ever experienced. I'm still trying to understand what the true safety feature of the emergency stop is.

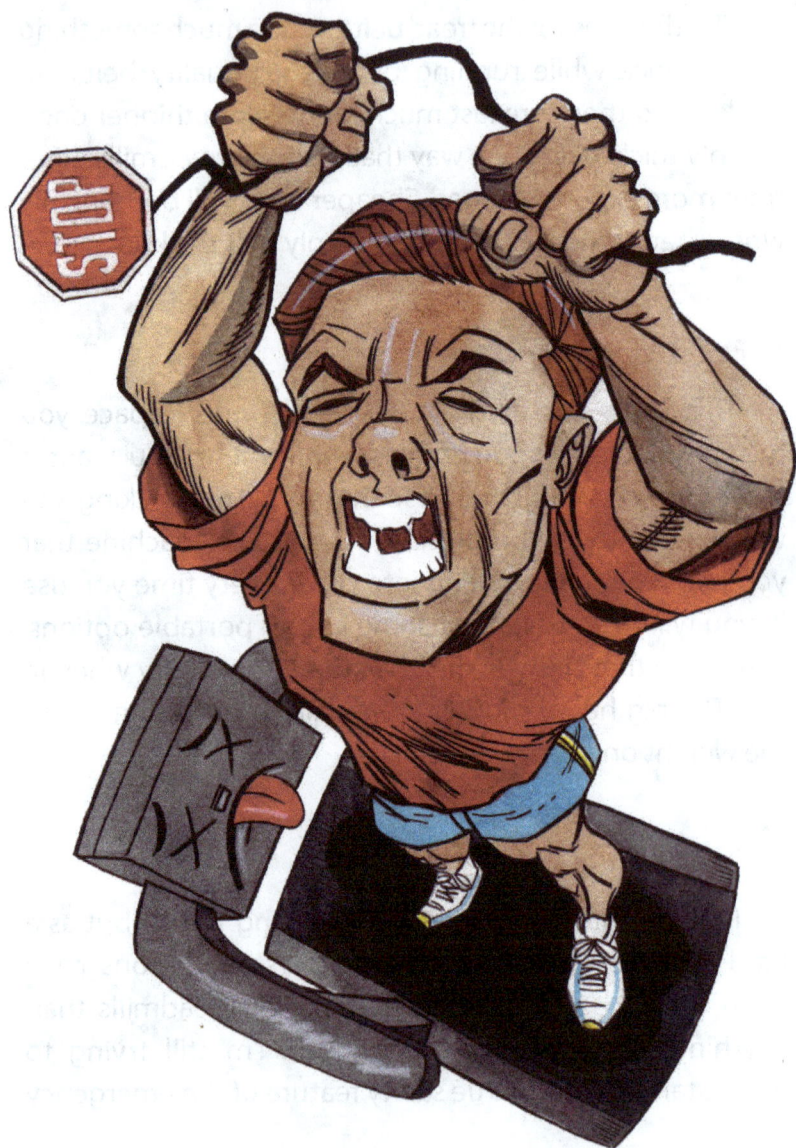

Short of causing friction burns if the belt rubs on your leg for a prolonged period of time if you've fallen, do you really care if the treadmill keeps running after you have fallen off? More importantly, how many people do you see actually hooking themselves up to the emergency cord? If you are a responsible and safety conscious person who does use these cords, then more power to you! Otherwise, you might want to look for an emergency stop that is simply not in the way or prone to accidental shut offs.

Things that DON'T matter (as much as a salesmen may lead you to believe):

1. Extended Warranty

I know it sounds counterintuitive to say that an extended warranty isn't worth it, but warranties are basically just insurance. If you buy a machine that is a trusted name with a good size motor that delivers a solid CHP, the chances of you needing to use the extended warranty are extremely low. Besides, the parts that you'll eventually need the coverage for are probably not covered in the warranty in the first place. If they are, beware of labour costs. I don't know of many, if any, service technicians that will do any kind of repairs for less than $500.

In reality, most machines will come with some kind of a warranty and the good treadmills already come with excellent warranties. For example Landice has a lifetime warranty for as long as you own the machine. Also, take a really close look at the details of the coverage and play out how things will go. Remember, a lifetime warranty on the frame doesn't mean a whole lot other than it will most definitely outlast the parts that are more costly to repair.

2. Deck Width

If you've ever looked back at your footprints in the sand or snow, you will find that you actually run within a very narrow pathway. So the only advantage of deck width is if you tend to wander side to side due to distraction. However if you are doing this, you'll eventually reach the edge anyway.

The following accessories can be convenient, but as you've read in the treadmill setup chapter, there are much better alternatives than having any of these features actually built into your treadmill which you will often pay more for!

3. Built-in Video Screens

Screens seem like a good idea, however, there's a good chance that the screen will be too close for comfort while running. Even runners with excellent form will have some degree of vertical movement which can create vertigo if you attempt to focus on an object so close. A video monitor is also an extra feature that can frequently malfunction as your treadmill ages.

4. Built in Fans

Treadmill fans rarely create much more than a slight breeze for the power they possess. Between the heat generated from the motor, the moving belt and your resulting perspiration, you are much better off investing in a commercial grade fan that you can position to your preference beside, or in front of, your treadmill. My personal preference is to have one on the side and one behind me to create a decent cross breeze.

5. Drink holders

Many drink holders built into the console are oversized to accommodate a variety of bottle sizes. The problem with this is that they often shake and rattle as you run and will either fall over or just annoy the heck out of you. I use mine to hold PC speakers as they are heavy and don't move. Others have bottle cages attached to some point on the frame. A better option than built in bottle holders is to have a portable, adjustable tray beside your treadmill that you can place your water, fuel and a few extra towels on. Portable trays can be purchased for between $10 and $30 and provide much more convenience for the amount of items that you can keep close while you are on the treadmill.

6. Towel holders

If it comes with one, great. If not, forget about it. You will probably end up quickly draping your towel over the middle of the display console or side bar anyway at some point in your run rather than take the time to drape it on a holder. As mentioned above,

Beware of treadmills that are built to sell rather than built to last!!

BASIC TREADMILL MAINTENANCE

Vacuum and De-clutter

Keeping the area around your treadmill clean serves more than one purpose. First, its way more inviting and appealing to work out in a clean and organized area. It really bugs me if I leave a mess from my previous run so I make a point of cleaning up after myself once my run is done which includes wiping my machine down and bringing my empty bottles upstairs.

Second, your treadmill has electronics and moving parts including bearings. If you don't keep the area around the treadmill clean, particularly if you have pets that shed, your bearings and belt can wear prematurely. If you've never taken the cover off of your motor, you might be surprised at how much dirt gets in there. Even if you're a clean freak, the moving parts create a degree of air intake and static that attracts dirt so take your cover off every few months and vacuum the motor area really well.

CAUTION!!

Please be sure to UNPLUG your treadmill before performing any maintenance in the motor area!!!

Sanitation

Wiping down the treadmill before and after your workout in a gym is a no brainer but wiping down your own machine is also important to maintain not only good hygiene, but also the look and life of your console finish and frame. Some of the frame is often constructed of exposed steel which will begin to rust if moisture is left to sit since your sweat is salty.

Whether your treadmill is newer and has sat for a while as a clothes rack or has logged some serious mileage, it's a good idea to do a quick periodic test (perhaps yearly).

You may have experienced running on other treadmills either at a local gym and had the sensation of working harder, or perhaps less! This often has to do with treadmills requiring calibration. They are machines with moving parts after all, and therefore will require calibration at some point in time.

This allows you to see if your treadmill is actually running at 5 mph or 8 km/h.

Calibration

The following self calibration strategy was submitted to me by Ultra legend, coach and occasional treadmill user Paul DeWitt: If you are going to do hard workouts on a treadmill and it has a good number of miles on it, or it's been sitting for years, it's a good idea to find out how accurate it is. If you are using a treadmill at the gym, this may be impossible but if you have one at home, you should do this every year or so. We've had ours for over 10 years and it has always been dead on, but each time we move I like to check it to be sure. Note that you can't make an inaccurate treadmill accurate. But, if you know that it is off by **x** amount, you can take that into account when running your workouts. It really helps to have a piece of white chalk and/or some tape for this calibration exercise.

1. Put a piece of white tape on one edge of the belt – this will be the starting point of your measurement. If you have your treadmill manual with specifications, you might have the exact length of your entire belt. If so, you can skip the belt measuring process.

2. Measure the length of the belt from the tape to as far as you can on the top of the belt and make a mark with your white chalk there. You'll have to turn the belt by hand to get the complete loop. Mine is 139.0 inches.

3. Figure out how many miles that is:

139 inches divided by 12 = 11.5833333333 feet. And divided by 5280 feet per mile, my belt is 0.002193813131313 miles in length. Next we'll compare the distance INDICATED by the treadmill panel with the actual distance the belt travels. For this, you should do the test at a typical speed you run. If the calibration is off, you can then repeat at a few other speeds to see if the error is linear or not.

4. For my example, I'm using 7.6 MPH (7:53 pace) shown on my panel.

5. Get the treadmill up to speed, and count the number of revolutions needed to go 0.25 miles. You may need somebody to help you watch both the panel readout and the tape mark. Repeat this step twice, and if the numbers are different, do it a third time and get the average.

6. For my treadmill, it took 114 revolutions to show 0.25 miles on the display.

7. So the actual mileage was 114 revolutions of the belt x 0.0021938131313 per revolution, or 0.250095 miles. The indicated mileage on the panel was 0.25. So, dividing 0.250095 by 0.25, I find that I am running 0.038% further than my treadmill's panel shows. For my purposes, that means my treadmill is dead on accurate, but if yours is off by more than a percent, you may want to take that error into account when working out.

APPENDIX 1
– TARGET HEART RATE CHART

*Keep in mind that this target heart rate chart is based on **estimates**, and nothing beats finding out what your true individual maximum heart rate is!

Target Heart Rate Chart (appendix)

This target heart rate chart can help you to train smart by finding which zones you should be in for your runs! Based on an age-graded formula and relative estimated projected maximum heart rate calculations, this chart provides you with recommended training zones for all of your runs within a well-balanced training program. Of course, you need heart rate monitoring capabilities to take advantage of this training approach.

Heart Rate Chart Navigation

Find your age in the left column below and refer to the estimated maximum heart rate as well as the low and high end of each training zone.

Age	Max HR	Easy/Recovery Zone		General Aerobic		Steady/Distance Race		Anaerobic Zone		Vo2 Max	
	*Estimated	Low End	High End	Low End	High End	Low End	High End	Low End	High End	Low End	High End
14	196	108	128	129	147	149	161	163	173	175	186
15	196	108	127	129	147	149	160	162	172	174	186
16	195	107	127	129	146	148	160	162	171	173	185
17	194	107	126	128	146	148	159	161	171	173	184
18	193	106	126	128	145	147	159	161	170	172	184
19	193	106	125	127	145	147	158	160	170	172	183
20	192	106	125	127	144	146	158	159	169	171	182
21	191	105	124	126	144	145	157	159	168	170	182
22	191	105	124	126	143	145	156	158	168	170	181
23	190	105	124	125	143	144	156	158	167	169	181
24	189	104	123	125	142	144	155	157	167	169	180
25	189	104	123	125	142	143	155	157	166	168	179
26	188	103	122	124	141	143	154	156	165	167	179
27	187	103	122	124	140	142	154	155	165	167	178
28	187	103	121	123	140	142	153	155	164	166	177
29	186	102	121	123	139	141	152	154	164	165	177
30	185	102	120	122	139	141	152	154	163	165	176
31	185	102	120	122	138	140	151	153	162	164	175
32	184	101	120	121	138	140	151	153	162	164	175
33	183	101	119	121	137	139	150	152	161	163	174
34	183	100	119	120	137	139	150	151	161	162	173
35	182	100	118	120	136	138	149	151	160	162	173
36	181	100	118	120	136	138	149	150	159	161	172
37	180	99	117	119	135	137	148	150	159	161	171
38	180	99	117	119	135	137	147	149	158	160	171
39	179	98	116	118	134	136	147	149	158	159	170
40	178	98	116	118	134	136	146	148	157	159	169
41	178	98	116	117	133	135	146	148	156	158	169
42	177	97	115	117	133	135	145	147	156	158	168
43	176	97	115	116	132	134	145	146	155	157	168
44	176	97	114	116	132	134	144	146	155	156	167
45	175	96	114	115	131	133	143	145	154	156	166
46	174	96	113	115	131	132	143	145	153	155	166
47	174	95	113	115	130	132	142	144	153	155	165
48	173	95	112	114	130	131	142	144	152	154	164
49	172	95	112	114	129	131	141	143	152	153	164
50	172	94	112	113	129	130	141	142	151	153	163
51	171	94	111	113	128	130	140	142	150	152	162

Age	Max HR	Easy/Recovery Zone		General Aerobic		Steady/Distance Race		Anaerobic Zone		Vo2 Max	
	*Estimated	Low End	High End	Low End	High End	Low End	High End	Low End	High End	Low End	High End
52	170	94	111	112	128	129	140	141	150	151	162
53	169	93	110	112	127	129	139	141	149	151	161
54	169	93	110	111	127	128	138	140	149	150	160
55	168	92	109	111	126	128	138	140	148	150	160
56	167	92	109	111	126	127	137	139	147	149	159
57	167	92	108	110	125	127	137	138	147	148	158
58	166	91	108	110	125	126	136	138	146	148	158
59	165	91	108	109	124	126	136	137	146	147	157
60	165	91	107	109	124	125	135	137	145	147	156
61	164	90	107	108	123	125	134	136	144	146	156
62	163	90	106	108	122	124	134	136	144	145	155
63	163	89	106	107	122	124	133	135	143	145	155
64	162	89	105	107	121	123	133	134	143	144	154
65	161	89	105	106	121	123	132	134	142	144	153
66	161	88	104	106	120	122	132	133	141	143	153
67	160	88	104	106	120	122	131	133	141	142	152
68	159	88	103	105	119	121	131	132	140	142	151
69	159	87	103	105	119	120	130	132	140	141	151
70	158	87	103	104	118	120	129	131	139	140	150
71	157	86	102	104	118	119	129	130	138	140	149
72	156	86	102	103	117	119	128	130	138	139	149
73	156	86	101	103	117	118	128	129	137	139	148
74	155	85	101	102	116	118	127	129	136	138	147
75	154	85	100	102	116	117	127	128	136	137	147

A few notes about some of the training zones above:

- The easy/recovery zones are for days that follow higher intensity runs such as a race, long run or speed work . Since the goal of this workout is recovery, it's important that the intensity is kept low to promote fresh blood flow (hyperemia) while minimizing further muscle damage. This is one of those zones that can be substituted with a day off!

- The general aerobic zone as that zone which will constitute most of your training.

- The steady/distance pace is typically a zone to avoid on a regular basis unless you are practicing marathon race pace. Otherwise, this zone is typically too fast for good aerobic development but too slow for effective anaerobic development. A.K.A. 'No-man's land'

- The anaerobic zone is stimulated through the successful execution of tempo runs. This zone should not be visited frequently in training unless you are experienced with it.

- The Vo2 max training zone is where your heart rate should reach during speed sessions such as intervals .

I sincerely hope that the application of the content in this book will help you to shift your outlook towards your training time on the treadmill from tolerance to enjoyment, and that you can appreciate them for the awesome training tools they really are.

Here's to your reliable training partner, always there to help, in your endless pursuit of setting and meeting your running goals!

DEREK LALONDE

www.ingramcontent.com/pod-product-compliance
Lightning Source LLC
Chambersburg PA
CBHW062055270326
41931CB00013B/3083